To Paul,

Thank you for the countless times you've made me crack up laughing and for being my safe harbour as I navigated through my own experiences, which have ultimately led to the stories and teachings in this book. And for showing me how to stop worrying about what other people think.

Powerful

Be the Expert in Your Own Life

Maisie Hill

GREEN TREE

LONDON · OXFORD · NEW YORK · NEW DELHI · SYDNEY

GREEN TREE
Bloomsbury Publishing Plc
50 Bedford Square, London, WC1B 3DP, UK
29 Earlsfort Terrace, Dublin 2, Ireland

BLOOMSBURY, GREEN TREE and the Green Tree logo are trademarks of
Bloomsbury Publishing Plc

First published in Great Britain 2024

For legal purposes the Acknowledgements on p. 214 constitute an
extension of this copyright page

A catalogue record for this book is available from the British Library

Library of Congress Cataloguing-in-Publication data has been applied for

ISBN: TPB: 978-1-4729-7892-9; ePUB: 978-1-4729-7893-6; ePDF: 978-1-4729-7894-3

2 4 6 8 10 9 7 5 3 1

Typeset in Minion Pro by Deanta Global Publishing Services, Chennai, India
Printed and bound in Great Britain by CPI Group (UK) Ltd, Croydon, CR0 4YY

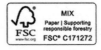

To find out more about our authors and books visit www.bloomsbury.com
and sign up for our newsletters

CONTENTS

INTRODUCTION

How does the idea of being powerful sit with you – do you feel comfortable with it? Is it something you yearn for, embrace with ease, or shy away from? Many of my clients want to feel powerful but at the same time, experience unease at the idea of it. And it's no wonder. Between harmful expressions of power such as authority and control over others, dominance and manipulation, power has become a dirty word.

But true power isn't predatory; it's purposeful. It's not about having control over others; it's about mastering oneself. Being powerful involves a quiet determination that drives us forward in our day-to-day lives; the intrinsic motivation that keeps us going even when the odds are stacked against us. It is the force we can connect with in order to assert ourselves. It is the inner strength that allows us to navigate life's uncertainties with courage and conviction, the resilience we harness when faced with adversity and the self-trust we find in moments of doubt.

Personal power is not about controlling external circumstances or people but about mastering our reactions to them. It connects us with our deeper purpose as well as understanding that we are the authors of our own narratives.

Being powerful necessitates that you be the expert in your life. Instead of seeking the opinion and permission of others, you will learn to trust your own intuition and judgement, listening to that inner voice that knows what is best for you, rather than being swayed by external pressures or expectations. With personal power, you recognise your own worth and are unafraid to advocate for your needs, desires and boundaries.

But that doesn't mean that you will always feel fantastic. I know how to coach myself and I'm excellent at it... I know how to work with my nervous system... I know my menstrual cycle intimately... I'm comfortable with a whole range of emotions... And I have meltdowns... Days when I feel sad, days when I feel massively challenged and days when I doubt myself and everything I've created. Of course I do. I'm human. These things don't go away just because you become an expert in them, but what changes is your capacity to have these experiences. This book will help you increase your capacity and build your resilience by finding ways to be *in* the challenge and discomfort while also being compassionate towards yourself.

I'm the founder of Powerful, a supportive life-coaching membership where women and non-binary folks from all over the world come together to learn how to silence their inner critic, tame the overwhelm and step into a life of clarity and confidence. If you've read my previous book, *Period Power*, you'll have learned how to harness your hormones and get your cycle working for you, but you may still need support with managing your mindset and stress responses, which is where this book comes in.

When I'm working with clients, I typically see people either opting out of things that are challenging or pushing themselves through something challenging by criticising themselves. Although they can do it, they've been mean to themselves throughout the process. And while there are times when it's 100 per cent necessary to skip things that are challenging to recover or protect yourself, it can turn into avoidance. Rather than increase your resilience and capacity, it decreases them.

Life will never be a neatly tied package. It'll throw curveballs and put obstacles in your path, from daunting decisions to unanticipated emotions and tricky conversations. Yet, as you'll discover within these pages, it's not about avoiding those challenges, but understanding and navigating them with grace, compassion and resilience, and appreciating that your reactions aren't marks of failure. Instead, they're signs that you're navigating a world filled with challenges, using the tools that millennia of evolution have handed down to you and a testament to the tapestry of experiences that have shaped you.

But you've got a new toolkit now. The chapters of this book aren't prescriptive solutions – they're perspectives that you can blend with your own. Viewpoints that, I hope, offer a clearer lens to see yourself through, a lens that's less judgemental and more accepting, because you aren't a problem that needs to be solved, nor are you broken. You're human and humans are inherently messy, complicated creatures. If you take anything from these pages, I hope that it's the idea that 'perfect' is a myth.

My Story

For most of my life, I struggled with my emotions. I would swing from feeling so full of emotion that it felt like I was going to explode to feeling completely numb and removed from the world. This is the book that I wish I'd had to help me navigate those times, because back in my teens and twenties I experienced spells of depression, and for many years, self-harming was how I 'handled' my feelings when they felt too much.

But it wasn't all shit, because this would alternate with the delicious, soaring highs that would come about when I was in the phase of my menstrual cycle where my hormones felt like they were for once on my side. Of course, at the time, I had no idea that my menstrual cycle was influencing me so much, because that's not what we were taught back then (my hope is that's changed since my first book, *Period Power*, came out).

Awareness of my menstrual cycle wasn't the only thing missing from my education and upbringing, though. Nobody taught me how to feel my emotions. Nobody told me that thoughts aren't factual and are therefore worth questioning. And nobody explained to me that my nervous system's stress responses were the reason why I would sometimes feel so irritated and worked up, or completely overwhelmed and stuck. Or for that matter, why I found it so hard to have boundaries and put a stop to my people-pleasing tendencies.

These are life skills that you probably weren't taught either, but, as I've discovered in my personal and professional life, it's never too late to get to know yourself like this. And I'm going to give you the information you need to understand yourself better; to make sense of your life through the lens of your nervous system, stress responses and hormones, and to appreciate how your mindset and emotions impact your experience of life.

This isn't about creating a perfect life or, indeed, a happy one. In fact, the whole point of this book is to show you that life is messy – and that's okay. By befriending your nervous system, bringing awareness to your mindset and any thought patterns that are unhelpful and, very often, self-destructive in nature, and learning how to experience your emotions so that you stop being terrified of them, you'll be able to give up the need to control the world around you. That means you'll be better able to experience the ups and downs of life.

Your Story

As you go about your day, reacting and responding to situations, other people and your environment, you may be overwhelmed by a whirlwind of emotions and thoughts. You may even find yourself descending into a shame spiral, recalling every negative comment you've ever received and criticising yourself for every misstep, every oversight. Before you know it, all your confidence has deserted you, you're doomscrolling to distract yourself and you feel awful.

I want you to be able to make sense of your reactions and responses, because without that awareness and understanding, the inevitable happens. Rather than seeing them for what they are, you assign meaning to your experiences and instead of seeing how your stress responses drive your behaviour, you tell yourself that you're incapable, unlovable and unworthy.

I'm going to help you stop doing that, because not only is it exhausting, but it's also holding you back. If you feel overwhelmed by stress, paralysed by perfectionism and fear of how others will react, or trapped in a never-ending cycle of people-pleasing, you're not alone. These reactions are not flaws or failures, they are inherent parts of our human wiring, shaped by millennia of evolution and the intricate dance of neurons and hormones.

In this book I'm going to give you the science that explains your everyday experiences. This knowledge will help you understand why you behave the way you do, so that you can navigate life with grace, resilience and self-love. You'll find a compassionate exploration of the challenges that everyone faces in some way, as well as the tools to overcome them. We'll review the physiology of stress and the natural defences of your nervous system and I'll guide you towards understanding, rather than judgement and shame.

We'll also explore the impact of female socialisation and how you can reclaim control over your emotions and decisions. You'll learn to trust yourself instead of beating yourself up. I'll gently remind you that you are enough, and I'll encourage you to build a more compassionate and respectful relationship with yourself, one that's rooted in self-acceptance rather than self-improvement.

This isn't a book that's designed to help you create a life where everything goes perfectly and challenges don't arise. As I've said earlier, life is messy. My aim is to help you be able to experience challenges, because within that messiness lies our humanity, our potential for growth, our chance to become strong, confident and capable.

This is a loving invitation to accept yourself, flaws and all, and to forge a path towards a more fulfilling and self-compassionate existence. You don't need to be fixed, because you aren't broken. You just need the tools that I believe we should all be taught early on in life. That's why I won't be giving you a prescriptive, rigid set of rules to follow either.

Through client case studies and practical insights, each chapter will enable you to understand that there are very understandable reasons why we *all* struggle with these things. You'll sigh with relief, embrace your humanness and discover simple and effective ways to change things.

In every group coaching session that I run, there will be a client who feels there's something wrong with them that needs to be fixed, but the truth is that for every person who gets coached on these issues, there are dozens of others on the call who are nodding their heads in recognition. These commonalities that bind us in our human experience have informed the way I teach, coach and now write. I've infused each chapter with the collective healing, wisdom and experiences that take place on my coaching calls.

My hope is that as you read them, you feel a loosening of inner judgement, criticism and shame. This is about adding layers of understanding and compassion to the complex web of stress responses, socialisation, emotions and behaviours that make you human. It's about empowering you to make sense of your reactions and responses without putting yourself down or exhausting yourself in the process.

When your internal world shifts, your experience of the world around you does, too. Imagine a life where you feel at home in yourself, where you can face the world with an unshakeable sense of self, ready to go out and do your thing. This book will empower you to do just that.

How to Read this Book

You have options. If a specific chapter calls to you, feel free to jump ahead. There's no right way to read this book. However, I encourage you to start by exploring how your nervous system operates in chapter 1. That way you can make sense of your responses to whatever's going on in your world. There's going to be some science involved, but this isn't a dry, textbook-style read. Throughout this book you'll encounter the inspiring stories of my coaching clients. Their journeys exemplify the transformative power of embracing these life skills. Together, we will delve the most common themes that I help my clients with as a life coach. From procrastination and perfectionism to defensiveness, boundaries and people-pleasing, each chapter holds the key to unlocking your inner power.

In each chapter we'll also tackle a specific challenge that you and countless others face every day. We'll unpick perfectionism and procrastination, and decipher the art of dealing with defensiveness, how to cope with criticism and the powerful world of personal boundaries. Along the way, you'll meet inspiring folks from my life coaching practice who've grappled with these challenges and made profound shifts in their lives.

Ultimately, I want you to feel at home in your body and in your mind. To be able to be you. To reduce the ways you criticise, judge and shame yourself. To stop over-apologising and over-explaining yourself. And to turn the dial way the hell up on your self-compassion. I know from experience that when you do that, your life will shift in ways that you can't even fathom right now.

Download Your Free Workbook

I've created a companion workbook to help you interact with the material on a deeper level, to personalise the strategies and to truly make them your own. Whether you're exploring your nervous system, wrestling with perfectionism, or setting new boundaries, the workbook provides a structured space for you to reflect, plan and dream.

To access your free workbook, simply visit: www.maisiehill.com/powerful-workbook

A note on language

I apologise to those of you who are neuroscientists. As an autistic person, I am very particular about using the correct terminology, but this isn't an academic textbook and I've chosen to keep the language and explanations accessible and applicable.

Chapter 1

Staying alive

You exist in a world that's full of threats. All day, every day, your body navigates a remarkable number of potential dangers to keep you alive. Even as you read these words – hopefully in a calm environment where you feel safe – your body is running software in the background that's constantly on the lookout for cues of danger and cues of safety. This software is your stress response system (SRS – make a mental note of the acronym because you'll come across it many times in this book) and it's time to get to know yours, because it's in charge of the whole damn show.

The SRS is the powerful combination of your nervous and endocrine systems. Your nervous system is a network of nerves that are responsible for regulating bodily responses, such as breathing and the rate at which your heart beats, all without you having to think about it. Your endocrine system is made up of glands that produce and release hormones, and together, as the SRS, they keep you alive.

Given that the SRS's job is all about survival, its responses will trump *anything else* you've got going on in your life. It takes in information from your environment, processes it and if it perceives a threat – real or imagined – it will initiate a stress response, and a set of behaviours, before you have the cognitive ability to recognise what's going on. However, my bet is that until you picked this book up, nobody had ever explained the significance of this to you, or at least not in a way that makes sense or is useful to you (don't worry, I've got you covered on that front).

Unfortunately, without the lens of understanding that comes from knowing your SRS, your mind will leap to other conclusions about your behaviour. When you walked away from a conversation or situation because you couldn't handle it, you might have thought that meant you're no good at commitments and it doesn't take much for you to leave. When you snapped at your partner, kid or a stranger on the bus, you might have concluded that you're highly strung, overly sensitive or just a terrible person. And what about those situations where you wanted to speak up, but found you couldn't? You probably made that mean something about you – that you lack courage and are a scaredy cat, for instance.

And let's be real, other people will have assigned meaning to your behaviour, too, just like you do when you're trying to make sense of their behaviour. This is what we do as humans, but I'm about to help you to understand your behaviour in a radically different way and it'll shine a light on why those around you behave in the way that they do as well. In doing so, my hope is that you'll treat yourself and others with way more compassion.

Really, Really Bad

We hear about how stress is really bad for us all the time and there is a mounting body of evidence that shows that stress *does* have negative consequences for our health and well-being (there's also evidence that says it really depends on how you frame the stress). However, it's important to remember that your innate ability to jump into a stress response is what's kept you alive. It's also what's enabled our species, not to mention a whole host of other organisms, to survive – birds, reptiles, fish, mammals and even bacteria use stress responses to stay alive, too.

Because the descriptions of stress that you and I would use tend to be along the lines of *feeling under pressure, overwhelmed* or *struggling to cope*, we tend to focus on how bad stress is and so neglect to remember its usefulness. From a medical perspective, stress responses also include defence responses such as fever and pain that are crucial when your body is combatting the invasion of bacteria or a virus or following an injury. Even coughing, vomiting and diarrhoea are protective mechanisms when the body is experiencing physical stress and suppressing them can lead to delayed recovery and medical complications. I'm going to leave that side of things to the doctors, though, and instead concentrate on the responses that you experience on a daily basis.

If you think back to your school science lessons, you may recall the phrase 'fight or flight', a stress response that's designed to protect you by getting you to defend yourself against danger or to run away from it. While most of us aren't in high-risk situations that require this level of response every day, your nervous system *is* being activated on the regular. Throughout this book, I'll be referring to these responses as they're going to help you make sense of the parts of your life that feel challenging, hard or even downright terrifying. Knowing what's happening and why is going to give you options and the ability to work with your SRS, instead of feeling you're a victim of it.

The Stress Response Symphony

Fight-or-flight stress responses are nothing short of amazing; they are so fast-acting that they allow you to react before you realise what's going on. When your nervous system perceives a real or interpreted threat in your environment, your SRS acts swiftly and with certainty. This is hugely advantageous, because when you encounter a threat, you don't want to waste precious time thinking, 'Oh look, that could be dangerous... Maybe I should do something... Should I hang around and fight or should I run away...? I think I should probably run away.' Needing to think like that to generate a response would slow you down considerably and drastically decrease your chances of survival.

Instead of this sluggish, thought-based way of doing things, your SRS leaps into action and takes the following steps:

1. The sensory systems of the brain evaluate potential sources of stress and relate them to your existing state, as well as your previous stressful experiences.
2. When a stressful challenge is detected, the brain activates your autonomic nervous system (ANS) – the division of your nervous system that, largely unconsciously, controls bodily functions. A branch of this is called the sympathetic adrenal medullary system (SAM), which uses hormones to increase essential bodily functions like blood pressure and the release of energy, while decreasing the ones that aren't essential at that moment, like digesting.
3. Simultaneously, the brain activates the HPA axis. This consists of three glands – the hypothalamus, pituitary and adrenals – it's where the nervous and endocrine systems intertwine, and it's responsible for the release of hormones that drive the fight-or-flight response.

This expertly coordinated sequence of events is kickstarted by the amygdala – a complex structure of cells found in the middle of the brain. Its name is derived from the Greek word *amygdale*, meaning almond, due to its almond-like shape, and you have one in each hemisphere of your brain. Historically, the amygdala is largely known as a threat detector and generator of fear to elicit a stress response, but more recent research has highlighted its involvement in motivation and reward processing.

By receiving information from the sensory systems of the body, the amygdala can detect potential threats in your surroundings before you're consciously aware that there's something to be fearful of. It's also involved in the formation of memories of fear-inducing events. Our understanding of the amygdala continues to evolve and it is now generally accepted that the amygdala plays a significant role in creating emotional responses not just to negative things in our environment, but to positive ones too.

The amygdala's next-door neighbour is the hypothalamus and there's a very good reason why these two are situated so close to one another. When the amygdala detects a potential threat, it immediately sends this information to the hypothalamus, which, in turn, triggers a hormonal cascade that includes the release of adrenaline and cortisol via the HPA axis. This swift response causes a number of reactions:

- Heart rate accelerates and blood pressure increases. That's why it feels like your heart is going to burst out of your chest and you can suddenly feel your blood pulsing through you.
- Blood sugar levels increase in order to provide the enormous amount of energy that's required to fight or run away.
- Breathing increases so that you can take on more oxygen.
- Digestion slows or stops altogether, because who needs to be using up energy digesting your lunch when your heart and lungs need all the energy they can get?
- Blood flow to the surface of the body is reduced, which is why people often pale when stressed (you can also flush as blood rushes to your head and brain).
- Blood flow to the muscles, brain, legs and arms also increases, because you're going to need them for running or defending yourself.
- Sweat cools the body and makes its surface slippery to aid escape.
- Muscular tension increases to provide extra speed, strength and endurance, and to guard against injury. That's why in stressful situations you *feel* tense, because your body is doing a great job of trying to protect

you. (We'll look at whether defending yourself is necessary and what to do if it isn't in chapter 3).

- Blood clotting speeds up to prevent excessive blood loss if you're injured.
- Tunnel vision and the temporary loss of hearing (auditory exclusion) can also occur under high stress, causing your field of vision to narrow and for sounds to become dulled or distant.
- Activation of the SRS not only prepares the body for immediate physical action, but also enhances cognitive functions related to threat detection and decision-making. The increased blood flow to the brain improves focus, alertness and the ability to quickly assess and respond to the situation at hand.

This is a response in which we feel highly activated and compelled to take action, and thank goodness for that, because how else would we summon all that's needed to flee or fight? Both options require an enormous burst of energy, which is why your experience of this state feels sudden and huge. After all, if you were out on the savannah and came across a predator, entering a state of hyperarousal that gets you moving is what's going to give you the best chance of survival.

Scared Stiff

The fight-or-flight response to a perceived threat relies on mobilisation and taking action, but there is a third response that involves a completely different strategy and that's *immobilisation*, aka the freeze response.

Just like fight or flight, freezing is an automatic, involuntary response. In a split second, your SRS decides that rather than run away or fight, the best option is to freeze while also being highly alert to what's going on around you, which is why it's sometimes referred to as *attentive immobility*. But whereas fight or flight is governed by the sympathetic branch of the nervous system, freezing occurs when both the sympathetic and parasympathetic branches of the nervous system are activated, and the parasympathetic branch dominates.

Orienting is a type of freeze response, the kind you might go into when something in your surroundings gets your attention and you're faced with a potential threat. It's what you might notice yourself doing when a sound startles you or a sudden movement demands your attention. Orienting slows you down so that you can scan your environment and orient yourself to whatever is going on, so that you can respond appropriately if necessary. It activates a state of hypervigilance that primes you for further nervous system response.

Freezing is the classic deer in the headlights' scenario, where an animal stands stock-still or plays dead, and it's what humans are encouraged to do, should they encounter a brown bear (rather you than me). Death-feigning is observed in several species, including rabbits, guinea pigs, chickens and swifts, as well many insects, snakes and frogs. They are all able to pretend they are dead to try and survive (the term 'playing possum' comes from the opossum's ability to feign death).

However, playing dead is risky and relies on the predator handling its prey differently if it thinks it's already dead – loosening its grip and thus providing an opportunity to escape – or leaving it alone altogether, because an animal that's already dead carries the risk of passing on an infection. Depending on the type of creature doing the freezing, they may also employ camouflaging techniques and even emit a foul-smelling substance to further the impression that they're already dead.

The freeze response isn't limited to physical immobility; it can also involve a sense of emotional or psychological immobility. In situations of intense fear or threat, we may feel emotionally frozen, unable to express or process emotions effectively.

Research suggests that the freeze response may serve as a defence mechanism in situations where escape or confrontation is not feasible. By remaining still and unresponsive, we hope to reduce our chances of attracting further attention or aggression from the threat. Freezing isn't a conscious choice or a sign of weakness. It's a physiological response deeply rooted in our evolutionary history. Understanding and accepting the freeze response can help individuals navigate and process their reactions to traumatic or stressful events.

Various factors influence the freeze response, including individual temperament, past experiences and the nature of the perceived threat. Some individuals may have a tendency to freeze more readily, while others may exhibit a stronger fight-or-flight response. In cases of trauma, the freeze response can become maladaptive or unhelpful if it persists beyond the immediate threat. This can lead to symptoms such as dissociation, numbing and difficulty in forming meaningful connections with others.

Why Didn't You Do Something?

Victims of crime are often asked, 'Why didn't you do something? Why didn't you run away or defend yourself?' Even in the absence of being asked this, they may berate themselves for not doing something, anything. But when the freeze response immobilises you, taking action and defending yourself simply aren't options for you.

This type of paralysis, known as *tonic immobility*, is an uncontrollable response to the presence of an extreme threat in which a person cannot say or do anything, because their movement and vocal responses are inhibited and are outside conscious control. It's only when they feel safe enough that these functions come back online.

In 2017, a Swedish study found that 69.8 per cent of women who had experienced sexual assault reported experiencing tonic immobility. Those that experienced it were more likely to have PTSD (post-traumatic stress disorder) at the time of the assault, which suggests the compounding effects of trauma – that experience of trauma can lead to further trauma. Those who experienced tonic immobility were also more likely to experience PTSD and depression six months later.

Tonic immobility is a reflex that leads to a state of paralysis and overrides any competing tendencies to take action. It's important to name this involuntary response because without this education, victims are more likely to blame themselves and be judged by others for not taking action in the way they wanted to, but were unable to.

Smoke Without Fire

Picture this: you're in your kitchen, making toast for breakfast. Suddenly, the smoke alarm goes off. There's no fire, just a bit of smoke from the slightly overdone toast, but the alarm doesn't know that, it's just doing its job, alerting you to potential danger. Your SRS is a lot like that smoke alarm. It's designed to protect you by alerting you to potential threats, so that you can take appropriate action. But just like the smoke alarm that can't tell the difference between a house fire and burnt toast, your SRS can't always distinguish between real threats and perceived ones, so it is activated more often than it needs to be. This is a very good thing, because even if nine times out of 10 it's being extra in its response, it only takes one occasion for it to get it wrong for things to end badly.

However, although we want the nervous system to err on the side of caution, there are more perceived threats than there are actual threats, and often we're having stress responses to situations that solely or largely exist in our minds. Thankfully, though, that means we have some control over our experience, which is what the subsequent chapters will help you with.

The problem is that if your SRS is being activated all the time or you're spending an excessive amount of time in stress responses, it costs a lot, because running the SRS involves trade-offs. In very simplistic terms, when your system is being flooded with stress hormones that will help you to survive, you're also using up a lot of energy. This is fabulous when you need to run away from a dangerous situation, but less so when you're just discussing a point of tension with your family or housemate.

If we were to make the SRS even more effective, the rate of stress-related diseases such as metabolic syndrome (a cluster of conditions that increase your risk of stroke, heart disease and type 2 diabetes) would be increased. On the other hand, if we decrease your stress responses, your likelihood of developing stress-related conditions would decrease, but so would your ability to handle stressful situations. So, like most bodily responses, a happy medium is best.

The good news is that just as we can learn to differentiate between a house fire and burnt toast, we can learn to manage our SRS more effectively. We can learn to recognise when our 'smoke alarm' is going off unnecessarily and to respond in a way that supports our well-being rather than exacerbating our stress.

Regulated/Dysregulated

Throughout this book, I'll use the terms *regulated* and *dysregulated* to describe the nervous system states. *Regulated* simply means feeling alright; not necessarily fantastic or particularly calm, but able to handle the ups and downs of your day. *Dysregulated* refers to stress responses such as fight, flight and freeze.

The Polyvagal Theory

In 1995, behavioural neuroscientist Dr Stephen Porges proposed a new understanding of the autonomic nervous system. Admittedly some aspects are still considered controversial, but in his polyvagal theory, Porges described three nervous system states that limit the range of behaviours and psychological experiences that are available to us. The first two states are fight/flight and freeze, and the third involves what he called the social engagement system (SES), an interaction system that allows mammals to interact and create bonds between one another.

In his proposed theory, Porges states that the SES emerged as the brain and cranial nerves developed, resulting in the ability to use the muscles of the face, head and neck that allow us to gesture, make eye contact and add intonation to our voices. If another person appears in your field of vision while you're reading this page, you might look up, especially if you're in an environment where you don't know the people around you, because your nervous system is continually picking up cues of threat and cues of safety, and so environments that are less familiar are more likely to require a degree of keeping an eye out.

However, even before your eyes leave the page, your nervous system is way ahead, rapidly assessing the cues coming from your surroundings, including the posture, expressions and tone of voice of those around you. You've probably had the experience of knowing that someone is watching you before your eyes have seen evidence of this – that's your nervous system at work.

As you look up, you begin to read those around you. Facial expressions that are relaxed, soft or warm in some way will help you to feel safe, whereas a grimace or scowl will create a very different response and bring the defensive mechanisms of fight, flight or freeze back online, because now there's something or someone to be wary of.

When the SES is operating, these defensive mechanisms are subdued. The nervous system continues to process information and evaluate potential threats, but it behaves like computer software: always running in the background, but ready to alert you to a potential threat. When the SES receives cues of safety, it cultivates calming behaviour that helps us to form positive attachments and social bonds.

Porges' polyvagal theory states that when the SES is online, the nervous system is in a regulated state, in which we feel safe, social and connected. Therefore the three nervous system states are:

Safe and social (aka ventral vagal)

When I say safe and social, I don't mean you at your dazzling best at a party, chatting to all and sundry. This has nothing to do with how happy or how social you are, or for that matter whether you're an introvert or extrovert. So, if it's not that, what is it? Nervous system geeks like me describe it as a felt sense of safety, one in which we simply feel okay and are able to be in the world; one that involves being connected to ourselves, to others and to the world around us.

We can observe this in other mammals, too. When there's no threat around them, they lie around, preen themselves and each other, and engage in other behaviours that are only an option for them when they feel safe. But as soon as there's a whiff of danger, they're on high alert. Then, when the threat has passed, they return to grooming, eating and mating.

Safe and social is where we want to spend most of our time, because it's a regulated state and, as we'll explore in the coming chapters, spending most of your time in dysregulated states (stress responses) has all sorts of negative consequences for your health, behaviour, mindset and relationships.

Fight or flight (aka sympathetic)

When you go into fight or flight mode, you experience a surge of energy and an urge to take action. This is a defensive response and so the organs, systems and body parts that will aid you in running away or fighting are activated.

Freeze (aka dorsal vagal)

In freeze mode, you are quite literally scared stiff. In the presence of a threat, you freeze and become immobile, but what your experience of this looks and feels like will vary. You may feel fatigued, dizzy or faint. You may go numb or check out in some way. Or you may disassociate – a term which describes the experience of disconnecting from yourself, your thoughts, emotions, memories and surroundings, as a way of your mind coping with stress.

This type of freezing feels like a collapse or shutdown of the system, whereas some experts have described a functional freeze, one in which we don't go limp and feign death, but instead tense up and freeze, so there is the arousal of the nervous system that we associate with fight or flight, but at the same time we experience a paralysis of sorts.

These nervous system states are *reflexive*, because they occur as reflex reactions to your environment. They also involve the vagus nerve.

The Vagus Nerve

This incredible nerve is technically not one, but two nerves; one which emerges from the right side of the brainstem and one which emerges from the left. The vagus nerve controls a vast number of bodily functions, including:

- Eye contact
- Facial expressions
- Ability to tune other people's voices in and out
- Voice production
- Sensation in the throat
- Swallowing
- Regulating the heart's rhythm
- Slowing the heart rate down
- Constricting the bronchi (the two tubes that act as passageways between your windpipe and lungs)
- Stimulating the production of stomach acid
- Controlling the involuntary muscles of the oesophagus (the tube that takes food from your throat to stomach), stomach, gallbladder, pancreas and small intestine, and stimulating peristalsis (a wave-like motion that moves food through the digestive tract) and secretions of the gastrointestinal tract.

That's impressive. For one nerve to be involved in so many bodily functions in so many regions of the body is incredible, and its ability to do this is down to its size, spread and complexity. In fact, it's so long that it wanders all the way from the brain down to the abdomen, which is why it's sometimes referred to as the *wandering nerve*.

Here's what I want you to know about the vagus nerve: Once you go into a freeze state, it takes a while for you to come out of it, because the composition of the vagus nerve means that it takes a while for the body to get going again: Around 80 per cent of its fibres carry information from the body to the brain and 20 per cent carry information from the brain to the body. This means that the body needs to come back online for the brain to have any say in what the body does, so your brain can be screaming at you to move, but your body is unable to obey its command.

Neuroception

Neuroception is a fascinating concept that sheds light on the intricate workings of the SRS. Also coined by Dr Stephen Porges as part of the polyvagal theory, neuroception refers to the subconscious detection and interpretation of cues from our environment that influence our physiological and emotional state. It's the body's way of evaluating whether a situation is safe, dangerous or potentially life-threatening, all before your conscious awareness kicks in.

It operates through the collaboration of various brain structures, including the amygdala, hypothalamus and ventral vagal complex. These regions work together to rapidly evaluate sensory information and determine the level of threat present in the environment. For instance, let's say you enter a dimly lit, unfamiliar room. Without consciously thinking about it, your body's neuroceptive mechanisms kick into gear: Neural pathways carry information from your sensory organs to the amygdala, which acts as an early warning system. The amygdala then quickly assesses the sensory cues, such as lighting, sounds and potential threats, and sends signals to activate the appropriate stress response.

Interestingly, neuroception operates on a continuum of safety, danger and threat to life. It's not a binary system, but rather a nuanced process that continuously evaluates the environment and adjusts our physiological and emotional states accordingly. This means that neuroception can be influenced by a range of factors, including past experiences, social cues and cultural context.

Porges and his colleagues have discussed the important role of neuroception in shaping our behaviours and responses, linking it to various aspects of social engagement, including the formation of trust, the regulation of emotions and the ability to connect with others. Understanding neuroception can provide valuable insights into how we perceive and respond to stressors in our daily lives, and the subconscious workings of our SRS. By becoming more attuned to our neuroceptive processes, we can develop a deeper awareness of our own stress responses and gain greater control over our reactions.

Plastic Fantastic

Whether you feel safe or not in any given situation is going to depend on a multitude of factors, such as:

- Your internal environment and the presence of any physical stressors
- The environment around you (temperature, sights, sounds and sense of space)
- Who's around you (and how you perceive what they're up to)
- Your thoughts about a situation
- What the rest of your day has been like
- Whether there are any other sources of perceived stress
- Where you are in your menstrual cycle
- Your reproductive life stage and hormone status
- A history of trauma or adverse childhood experiences (ACEs – see pages 49–50)
- How your nervous system has been configured during the course of your existence
- How your ancestors' nervous systems were wired in their lifetimes.

Your experiences in the womb began to mould your SRS and it has developed over your lifetime, but even before you were a collection of cells, the experiences that shaped the nervous systems of your ancestors also informed the development of yours. What's crucial to understand, though, is that however your nervous system has been configured, you can rewire it.

Neuroplasticity is the ability of the nervous system to modify itself, both in terms of its structure and behaviour, in response to new information gleaned from experiences, sensory stimulation, development, damage and injury. That means that in every situation where you feel hijacked by stress responses, and feel defensive, anxious, fearful or worried, there are opportunities for you to reconfigure your nervous system. In doing so you'll stretch your nervous system, helping it to grow and form new neural connections, which, in turn, will increase your capacity for these experiences – to be in them without jumping into the extremes of fight, flight and freeze – and build resilience.

Neural loops and pathways

Your brain houses a mind-blowing 86 billion neurons. These nerve cells create an intricate landscape of neural loops and pathways that play a crucial role in shaping our responses to stress. These networks work together to transmit and process information, influencing how we perceive and react to the world around us. By understanding the dynamics of these neural loops, we can gain insight into the mechanisms behind the SRS.

Stress can impact the structure and functioning of these neural loops and pathways. Chronic stress can lead to alterations in the brain's architecture, affecting areas involved in emotion regulation, memory processing and decision-making. The repeated activation of the SRS reinforces neural pathways associated with stress, making it easier for our brains to perceive and react to potential threats. One key area of interest is the amygdala, the almond-shaped structure nestled deep within our brains. The amygdala acts as a crucial hub in the SRS, processing emotional and fear-related information. Studies have revealed that chronic stress can lead to increased amygdala activity, enhancing its sensitivity to potential threats. This heightened activation can contribute to the amplification of stress responses and the development of anxiety-related disorders.

Another significant player in the neural orchestra is the prefrontal cortex, the region responsible for higher-order cognitive functions such as decision-making and impulse control. Chronic stress has been found to impair the prefrontal cortex's ability to regulate emotional responses effectively, resulting in difficulties managing stress, as well as a greater susceptibility to impulsive behaviours and emotional reactivity.

The interplay between the amygdala and the prefrontal cortex is central in modulating stress responses. A healthy balance between these regions allows for adaptive regulation of emotions and the ability to flexibly respond to stressors, but chronic stress can disrupt this delicate balance, leading to an overactive amygdala and an underactive prefrontal cortex.

Understanding these neural loops and pathways offers us an insight into potential avenues for stress management and resilience-building. Through studying practices such as mindfulness meditation, researchers have found evidence of neural plasticity, the nervous system's ability to modify itself in response to experience and injury; your brain can rewire itself. Mindfulness-based interventions have been shown to strengthen connections between the prefrontal cortex and the amygdala, promoting greater emotional regulation and reducing stress reactivity.

But it's not just meditation that improves neural functioning. Studies have highlighted the positive impact of physical exercise, too. Regular exercise is associated with increased neuroplasticity, bolstering connections within the prefrontal cortex and enhancing its capacity to modulate stress responses. Engaging in activities such as aerobic exercise, yoga or even a brisk walk can provide not only physical benefits, but also support the development of neural pathways that promote resilience to stress. This is why anytime I know I'm going to be working on a project that is likely to stretch me, I prepare for it by using kettlebells and taking walks along the beach.

Our brains are malleable and capable of change. By increasing awareness of our stress responses, practising mindfulness and engaging in activities that support neural well-being, we can nurture the growth of adaptive neural pathways and enhance our ability to navigate stress with resilience.

Igniting Neural Firing

Neural firing refers to the electrical impulses that surge through interconnected neurons, transmitting information and facilitating communication within the brain. When we encounter a stressor, whether it be a looming deadline or a challenging situation, a cascade of neural firing is set in motion. This firing activity occurs in specialised regions, including the amygdala, hippocampus and prefrontal cortex, which, as you now know, are key players in processing emotions, memory formation and decision-making.

The amygdala, known for its role in processing fear and emotional responses, plays a vital part in initiating the stress response. Neural firing within the amygdala sends rapid signals to other brain regions, alerting them to the presence of a potential threat. This rapid activation sets the stage for a coordinated stress response, mobilising the body for action.

Simultaneously, the hippocampus, a region involved in memory formation and contextual processing, is engaged. The hippocampus acts as a kind of memory hub, consolidating information about the stressor and its associated context. This neural firing activity allows for the integration of new experiences into existing memory networks, providing a foundation for future responses to similar stressors.

Imagine you're preparing for an important presentation at work. As you gather your thoughts and organise your slides, your hippocampus is hard at work, orchestrating the neural firing activity that will help you remember crucial details. It's like a diligent librarian, cataloguing information about the presentation, the context in which it will take place and even your emotional state during the preparation process. When the time comes to deliver the presentation, your hippocampus taps into those stored memories, seamlessly integrating them into your conscious awareness. The neural firing patterns that were established during the preparation phase facilitate a smooth retrieval of information, ensuring you can confidently navigate your way through your slides and address questions from the audience.

The hippocampus' role in consolidating stress-related memories goes beyond just the presentation itself. It also helps link the experience of preparing and delivering the presentation to past experiences and emotions. For example, if you've successfully handled similar high-pressure situations in the past, the hippocampus retrieves those memories and integrates them into your current stress response. This integration provides a foundation for adaptive responses to future stressors, as your brain draws upon previous experiences to guide your actions and regulate your emotions.

The prefrontal cortex, the brain's executive control centre, also undergoes intricate neural firing patterns during the stress response. This region is responsible for higher-order cognitive functions, such as decision-making, impulse control and emotional regulation. If you're driving in heavy traffic and feeling stressed because you're trying to get to an important appointment on time, the stress of the situation triggers neural firing in your prefrontal cortex, the brain's executive control centre. Like a skilled conductor, the prefrontal cortex orchestrates the activity of different regions of your brain, ensuring a harmonious response to the stressor.

As you navigate the traffic, the prefrontal cortex engages in neural firing patterns that support your decision-making abilities. It helps you evaluate the available options, weighing up the benefits and risks of different routes and strategies. By inhibiting excessive activation of the amygdala, the prefrontal cortex prevents an overwhelming flood of stress responses, allowing you to maintain a level-headed approach to the situation.

The prefrontal cortex also aids with impulse control, preventing impulsive and potentially risky behaviours in response to the stress of being stuck in traffic. It's what hopefully enables you to resist the temptation to aggressively cut off other drivers or engage in road rage, promoting more adaptive and socially appropriate responses, all while regulating your emotions, so you stay calm and composed despite the frustrating traffic situation.

Chronic or prolonged stress can disrupt the delicate balance of neural firing dynamics. Research suggests that chronic stress can lead to hyperactivity within the amygdala, resulting in exaggerated fear responses, and increased vulnerability to anxiety and mood disorders. Additionally, chronic stress can impair neural firing patterns in the prefrontal cortex, compromising its ability to regulate emotions and make sound decisions.

Understanding the intricacies of neural firing opens up possibilities for interventions aimed at restoring balance and promoting resilience in the face of stress. Practices such as mindfulness meditation and cognitive-behavioural therapies have been shown to modulate neural firing patterns, promoting greater connectivity between regions involved in emotional regulation and executive control. These interventions can help recalibrate neural firing dynamics and support adaptive responses to stressors.

Past Meets Present

The impact of our ancestors' nervous systems on our own stress responses is a captivating area of study that highlights the interconnectedness of generations. Research in the field of epigenetics has revealed that the experiences and environments of our ancestors can influence the functioning of our own nervous systems, including our stress responses.

Epigenetics refers to the study of changes in gene expression that occur without alterations to the underlying DNA sequence. These changes are influenced by various factors, including environmental exposures, lifestyle and, yes, even those experiences of previous generations. It suggests that our genetic material is not solely responsible for determining our traits and behaviours; it interacts with the environment and can be influenced by our ancestors' experiences.

Studies have shown that traumatic experiences endured by previous generations can leave a biochemical mark on their DNA, potentially leading to changes in stress response regulation. Research conducted by Dr Rachel Yehuda and her colleagues examined the descendants of Holocaust survivors and found alterations in stress hormone regulation and increased prevalence of stress-related disorders, such as post-traumatic stress disorder

(PTSD). These findings demonstrate the impact of traumatic events being passed down through generations, shaping the physiological responses of subsequent offspring.

The effect of stress can extend beyond an individual's lifetime and impact future generations. Research on animals has provided insights into transgenerational effects on stress responses. In experiments involving rodents, exposure to stressors in one generation resulted in altered stress responses and behaviours in subsequent generations, even in the absence of direct exposure to stressors.

The mechanisms underlying these transgenerational effects are still being explored, but it's thought that epigenetic modifications, such as DNA methylation and histone modifications, play a role in transmitting the influence of ancestral experiences to subsequent generations. These modifications can impact gene expression patterns, ultimately influencing the functioning of the nervous system and stress response regulation.

While the impact of ancestral experiences on our nervous systems is significant, it's important to note that it does not determine our destiny. Helpfully, the field of epigenetics also highlights the potential for resilience and the capacity for change. Our experiences and environment can interact with our genetic predispositions to shape our stress responses. Considering the interplay between our ancestors' experiences and our own nervous system functioning provides valuable insights into the complexity of our stress responses, and reminds us that our biology is shaped by more than just our individual experiences.

Okay, now that you've got to know that beautiful nervous system of yours, let's take a look at the situations that feel challenging. You ready? Let's do this.

Chapter 2

Procrastination

When was the last time you procrastinated? Was there something you were meant to do today that you could have done, but didn't? Perhaps you're even reading this chapter as a sneaky way of avoiding doing that thing that you know you ought to. Procrastination is the act of voluntarily delaying and postponing tasks – often leaving them to the last minute or long past their deadline – despite your best intentions and your awareness of the potential negative consequences of doing so.

Procrastination is a term often misunderstood and misinterpreted. It's easy to label it as mere laziness and both terms carry the same harsh judgements: that if you could stop being so lazy and get it together, then it would all be alright; that if you were more organised then this wouldn't be an issue; that if you only had the mental fortitude to push through and get it done, everything would fall into place. But this perspective is not only unhelpful, it's also untrue. Procrastination is not a sign of personal failure or a unique flaw that only you possess. It's a universal human experience. Even the most organised, efficient and determined individuals have moments of procrastination. It's not a 'you' problem, it's a 'we' problem. So let's start by acknowledging that we all procrastinate and remove the self-deprecating narrative that often accompanies it.

Ironically, despite this being the second chapter, it's the last one I'm writing. Yes, I have been procrastinating about it. Or at least that's what a voice inside my head has been trying to tell me. Thankfully, I know not to indulge it, and I can counteract it with a far kinder and more helpful narrative, which is what I'm going to teach you how to do, too. Beating yourself up about not doing something rarely results in you doing it and, on the odd occasion that it does, it also fuels the fire of negative self-talk and the cycle of blaming and shaming yourself.

Giving In to Feel Good

If procrastination isn't a result of laziness or being disorganised, then what is it? Procrastination is a failure to self-regulate your emotions. It arises when we're confronted with tasks we'd rather not do – tasks that seem frustrating, pointless, boring or challenging. These tasks don't exactly inspire enthusiasm. Instead, they trigger a desire to avoid the discomfort they bring, leading us to procrastinate.

Researchers Dianne Tice and Ellen Bratslavsky encapsulated this phenomenon in the phrase 'giving in to feel good.' This strategy, however, provides only temporary relief – you may successfully dodge an uncomfortable emotion in the moment, but the longer-term consequences are far more distressing. The negative outcomes of not completing a task on time – or not completing it at all – can lead to feelings of shame or embarrassment.

The burden doesn't just get postponed to the future; it also grows. Even if there are no tangible negative consequences – say, the project gets delayed so the tasks that you were assigned don't seem to matter for the time being – the internal turmoil that unfolds over time can be significant. The negative self-talk, stress responses and harmful behaviours that result from procrastination can create a snowball effect, amplifying the discomfort far beyond what the initial task would have caused.

Procrastination is a battle between immediate comfort and future accomplishment. We dodge tasks that seem daunting, tedious or uninteresting, seeking instant relief in the form of delay. The reality is, most meaningful endeavours involve some degree of discomfort. Whether it's the mental effort of solving a complex problem, the emotional challenge of handling a difficult conversation, the physical strain of pushing our bodies to new limits or sending a short email that risks pissing someone off, growth often demands that we step outside our comfort zones.

The short-term comfort of procrastination comes with a hefty price tag. In borrowing against your future time and energy, interest accrues in the form of stress, guilt and negative self-perception.

The Watcher

Anytime that you realise you're procrastinating, ask yourself why. There will be a specific, or perhaps multiple, reasons why you're holding off on taking action, and the trick is to hone in on the reason behind it. This requires two skills: Being honest with yourself and becoming aware of your thoughts.

One of the first things I teach my clients is to 'become the watcher', a technique that simply means noticing your thoughts, emotions, reactions, responses and behaviours. Rather than simply reacting to everything that happens over the course of your day, you watch yourself and notice things – you are the watcher of your mind.

This creates some distance from your experience and with that comes perspective. When you have perspective, you can get curious about why you do things the way you do – not because there's anything wrong with it, but because awareness gives you choice. Becoming the watcher is all about noticing yourself and giving yourself options.

So why have I been delaying writing this chapter? I've been asking myself the same question and as I've become aware of my thoughts about writing it, I've observed a dominant and recurring sentence: *I don't know where to start*. This simple sentence, seemingly harmless, has been the root of my procrastination, leading me to feel confused and unsure – hardly the emotions that would propel me into taking action.

What's your sentence? Think back to the last thing you procrastinated on or something that feels significant from recent years. Can you find the sentence that was in your head that caused you to delay or put that task off? I've put you on the spot here, so if your brain is scrambling to pinpoint the reason behind your delay, take a moment and give it your best guess. Why did you delay taking action on that occasion? Here are my best guesses:

- I don't know where to start
- It won't take me long, so I'll just do it later
- It'll take ages, so I'll do it when I have more time
- I don't know what I'm doing
- I'm too tired
- I'm confused
- It'll be boring
- What I do won't be good enough
- I'm not good enough
- If I get it wrong, then I'll be in trouble
- If I get it wrong, then everyone will laugh
- People will think that I'm _____
- Everyone will realise that I'm _____

Negative self-talk like this feels like crap, so it's no wonder that our minds often choose to avoid the task at hand rather than endure such self-criticism, especially if instead of doing the task you need to do, you do something that releases dopamine and feels pleasurable instead, like scrolling on your phone or snacking. This avoidance is a form of self-protection, an attempt to escape the discomfort these thoughts bring, but of course it isn't protective in the long-run.

Your Perception of Procrastination

It's not just the thoughts that lead to procrastination that are worth paying attention to. What are your thoughts about being someone who procrastinates? When I'm coaching a client, I'm always interested in what they make it mean about themselves, because there's usually a hefty pile of shame that they're unsuccessfully trying to outrun. Sometimes the issue isn't procrastination, but your response to it. How you perceive and respond to these signals can make a significant difference in the degree to which it impacts your life.

If, like many of my clients, you view procrastination as a personal failing or as evidence that you're lazy or incompetent, then it becomes a source of shame and self-criticism. This negative self-talk only exacerbates anxiety and fear, leading to a vicious cycle of procrastination. Similarly, if you view your fear responses as signs that you're weak or cowardly, then you could feel embarrassed or guilty and try to suppress these responses, which can lead to additional stress and anxiety.

I don't know a single human who doesn't do it in some form – and that includes myself. Even the most organised, efficient and determined people I know do it. Really let that sink in. Everybody does it. It's not a *you* thing. You are not uniquely flawed. On this front, you are the same as everyone else, so let's start off with accepting that we all do it and remove the layer of 'I'm a no good, lazy, terrible human' that clouds procrastination.

Procrastination isn't inherently problematic, it's a natural human behaviour. Sure, it has negative consequences. However, I suspect that your response and thoughts about the act of procrastinating create more of an issue than if you just accept it and move on, so try to shift your perspective: accept that this is a thing all humans do and approach it with self-compassion and curiosity rather than judgement.

Procrastinating Perfectionism

Perfectionism, often disguised as a virtue, is a silent saboteur. Perfectionism is a trait that's characterised by striving for flawlessness and perfection, accompanied by critical self-evaluations and concerns regarding others' evaluations. It's a trait that's more prevalent than you might think, affecting up to 30 per cent of the population, with a higher prevalence among women. It's often associated with high levels of stress, anxiety and depression, and can even impact the formation of close relationships due to fear of judgement or rejection.

Many of my clients, particularly those who identify as high-achievers, don't realise that they're prone to perfectionism, because we typically associate perfectionism with a polished, manicured appearance and a tidy, organised lifestyle. However, perfectionism is not about outward appearances, high standards or striving for excellence, but rather an unrelenting pursuit of flawlessness, often accompanied by harsh self-criticism and concerns about others' evaluations of you.

Client Story

This is how my client Roxy describes her experience of perfectionism and procrastination: 'I always had high expectations of myself, but because I was stuck in avoidance and procrastination I didn't think of myself as a 'perfectionist'. I only did things last minute under intense stress and pressure, but in a way this was 'safe' as I never needed to find out whether I would produce the results I would actually be proud of if I gave myself more time. What I didn't realise was that I was constantly stuck in overwhelm, with a shut-down nervous system. It made my student era hellish and made me feel very dissatisfied and insecure about my career, never finding fulfilment and never feeling in control.'

With perfectionism, we set unreasonably high expectations for ourselves and are overly critical of our performance, even when it's gone fantastically. We ruminate over mistakes and try to hide them from others. This is accompanied by a constant sense of urgency and stress, all of which lead to a need to control, overworking, having little spare time and cycling between high achievement and exhaustion.

Here's a list of traits and behaviours that often manifest under the umbrella of perfectionism. If you find yourself nodding along to these, you might be prone to procrastinating perfectionism:

- Procrastination and paralysis: You delay starting or finishing tasks due to the fear of not being able to meet your own high standards or fear of how others will respond if it's not up to scratch.
- A sense of urgency and stress: You feel a constant need to rush, especially when it comes to acquiring new skills or qualifications.
- High expectations: You set the bar incredibly high for yourself and others, often unrealistically so.
- Overly critical of yourself: You tend to focus on your flaws and failures, rather than your strengths and successes.
- Rumination: You obsess over past mistakes or future challenges, often leading to anxiety and stress.
- Hiding mistakes: You go to great lengths to cover up errors, because they feel unbearable to you.
- Limited spare time: Your schedule is packed with tasks and responsibilities, leaving little room for relaxation – even activities that could be rejuvenating aren't because of how you approach them.
- Cycling between high-achievement and exhaustion: You push yourself to achieve, often at the cost of your physical and mental health.
- Absence of joy and fun: You're so focused on your goals and what needs to be done that you forget to enjoy the journey.
- Need to control: You feel a strong need to control your environment and the people around you, even when it's not necessary or beneficial.
- Defensiveness: You struggle to accept constructive criticism and often react defensively when your work is critiqued.
- Inflexibility: You struggle with change and have a hard time adapting to new situations or plans.
- Driven by fear: Your pursuit of perfection is more about avoiding failure and criticism than achieving success.
- Tasks take longer than necessary: You spend more time on tasks than required, not because you underestimate the effort, but because you're striving for perfection.

- Overworking is normal: You regularly work long hours and take on too many tasks, often without realising that you're overdoing it (and you probably have a very low tolerance for when other people point this out to you and suggest you take it easy).

Perfectionism is our brain's misguided attempt to keep us safe. It convinces us that if we can just do everything 'right' we can avoid criticism, judgement and failure. In reality, though, this mindset often leads to procrastination, as the fear of not being perfect can be paralysing. Understanding the connection between procrastination, perfectionism and mindset is the first step towards overcoming your own delaying tactics.

Client Story

Making that link between being a perfectionist and a procrastinator really helped my client Sarah: 'I was a people-pleaser and a perfectionist. I would always say yes to things. It led me to procrastination, but now that I know about stress responses, I recognise it as freezing and withdrawing. Now I realise when I'm dysregulated in my nervous system, but before I would have just thought I was being moody, which I attribute to how I've been socialised as a woman. I now recognise how important I am and that I can put myself first, and am learning the best way to support myself without being my biggest critic. I was always waiting or asking others for opinions, and now I do thought work and go for what I want! No more sitting in indecision. I recognise that I feared failure, but it is absolutely fine to fail. In fact, I would encourage everyone to fail – it's not as scary as you think and you will learn from it!'

Thought work

Thought work is a self-coaching technique that I teach my clients. It's the practice of becoming aware of what you think and how your thoughts impact how you feel and the actions that you take as a result. It emphasises the impact our thoughts have on shaping our reality.

Never Say Never

Have you ever noticed how starting out with a negative thought like, 'I won't do this well enough' not only causes you to procrastinate, but also escalates into finding a load of evidence of how you *always* procrastinate and *never* get anything done? This tendency to overgeneralise is a type of cognitive distortion; an exaggerated or irrational thought pattern that distorts your perception of reality, often leading you to view things as much more negative than they actually are.

We all do this from time to time, because it's part of the human experience, but when this negativity creeps into more and more of your internal dialogue and external conversations, it can contribute to an increasingly negative outlook and perception of yourself. Let's take a closer look at some common cognitive distortions:

- Over-generalisation: Using words such as 'always', 'never', 'everything' and 'nothing' in your thoughts and conversations.
- Polarisation: Seeing things in extremes with no middle ground (see page 41) – also known as 'all or nothing' or 'black and white' thinking.
- Personalisation: Believing you're responsible for things outside your control, leading to unnecessary emotional distress.
- Jumping to conclusions: Making negative, often extreme, predictions about what others will think or what will happen without sufficient evidence.
- Catastrophising: Imagining the worst possible outcomes in a situation, often starting with 'what if' doom and gloom scenarios (see page 146 for my favourite technique for handling this).
- Discounting the positive: Saying someone has only complimented you because they want something or, when you achieve something, telling yourself it's no big deal, because anyone could have done it.
- Blaming: Assigning guilt or responsibility for how you feel to someone else. For example, 'You're making me feel inadequate/guilty/bad.'
- Should-ing: Making statements with 'should' in them that cause you to experience emotions such as worry, fear, anxiety or guilt.
- Control fallacy: Believing your life is controlled by factors inside or outside of your control, leading to negative emotions such as helplessness and frustration.

- Fallacy of change: Assuming others should change to suit your needs or desires, and that they just need to be encouraged or pressured enough, often leading to disappointment and resentment.
- Emotional reasoning: Believing that what you feel must be true. For example, if you feel stupid, then you believe you must be stupid – like saying, 'I feel it, therefore it must be true.'
- Labelling: Assigning labels to yourself or others based on a single characteristic or event. For example, if you make a mistake, you might label yourself a failure or loser.
- Mind-reading: Assuming you know what others are thinking or feeling without any evidence, as though you've suddenly developed psychic abilities, but – spoiler alert – you haven't.
- Fallacy of fairness: Feeling resentful, because you think you know what's fair, as if you're the self-appointed judge and jury of fairness in the world, but other people don't agree with you.
- Negative filtering: Focusing almost exclusively on the negative aspects of a situation while ignoring any positive elements – like you've got a pair of negativity-tinted glasses on.
- Always being right: Believing your opinions are facts and are therefore correct, and in doing so failing to consider other perspectives and experiences – much as it pains me to say it, I'm not always right, and neither are you!

Recognising these cognitive distortions is not about providing more ammunition for self-criticism. Don't make the presence of them in your life mean anything about you, because they're something we all do. Instead, it's about gaining awareness of these thought patterns and understanding their impact on your behaviour. The more you observe your mind, the more familiar you'll become with your habitual thoughts, responses, emotions and behaviours. This awareness is a crucial step towards adjusting your thinking and overcoming procrastination. Remember, the goal is not to beat yourself up, but to empower yourself to take the actions you want to take.

Don't Neglect the Basics

Tiredness, whether due to lack of sleep or other factors such as overwork or stress, can also contribute to procrastination. Sleep deprivation impairs executive functions, which are crucial for self-regulation, making decisions and prioritising tasks to overcome procrastination.

Stress levels also play a significant role in procrastination. On the one hand, stress and the pressure of a deadline can be incredibly motivating. A moderate level of stress can be productive, creating enough arousal to take action. However, it can reach the tipping point where it becomes too much, leading to overwhelm and preventing you from taking any action at all. When stress levels are too high, cognitive functions such as decision-making and problem-solving can be impaired, making tasks seem more daunting and leading to avoidance behaviours. Feeling overwhelmed is associated with the freeze response and what I refer to as ostrich mode (see pages 143–4), so it's worth considering if you're procrastinating, or if what's being highlighted is a need to switch off and recharge your reserves.

If you're already feeling stressed, your instinct might be to push harder, to try and force yourself to take action, but this approach can exacerbate the problem. Sometimes, what you really need is to hit pause and intentionally rest. That doesn't necessarily mean lying down or taking a nap, although these can be excellent strategies when we're feeling overwhelmed or burnt out. When you find yourself unable to focus, instead of busying yourself with organising your inbox or another task, consider taking a short or more substantial break. If you've been sitting, get up and move. Simple adjustments, such as changing your posture, stretching, stepping outside or standing next to a well-lit window, or drinking some water can all give you what you need in the moment. Just be mindful you don't end up using them as excuses or forms of distraction.

Executive Functioning

Executive functioning refers to a set of cognitive skills that are required for managing and regulating our thoughts, actions and emotions. These skills include planning, decision-making, problem-solving, impulse control and the ability to switch focus between tasks. They are primarily managed by the prefrontal cortex, a part of the brain that is involved in complex cognitive behaviour, personality expression, decision-making and moderating social behaviour.

When it comes to procrastination, executive functioning plays a significant role. Procrastination, at its core, is a failure to regulate our behaviour and emotions effectively. We know what we should be doing, but we struggle to make ourselves do it. This disconnect between knowing and doing can be related to poor executive functioning skills, which is linked with autism and ADHD.

For instance, if we struggle with planning and decision-making, we might find it difficult to break down a large task into manageable steps, leading us to feel overwhelmed and avoid the task. If we struggle with impulse control, we might find it hard to resist the temptation to do something more enjoyable or less challenging, leading us to procrastinate about the task at hand.

Executive functioning skills are also crucial for managing the emotions associated with procrastination. They allow us to regulate our fear and anxiety, to shift our focus from the immediate discomfort of the task to the long-term benefits of completing it, and to develop strategies for managing our procrastination effectively.

The good news is that executive functioning skills are not fixed. They can be improved with practice and training using techniques that require planning, cognitive-flexibility, perseverance and problem-solving. Stress impairs executive function, so anything that reduces stress levels such as mindfulness practices and cognitive behavioural therapy can be useful, and mindful movement activities such as traditional martial arts, qi gong, tai qi and yoga have been shown to enhance executive functioning and could potentially help in reducing procrastination. Drawing on these approaches, I've developed a set of techniques that I teach to my clients. I encourage you to give them all a go, but feel free to pick and choose as they may not all be right for you.

Understanding procrastination as a failure to self-regulate emotions can provide valuable insights into why we procrastinate and how we can overcome it. My first suggestion isn't going to feel great, but here it is…

Embrace the suck

I told you it wouldn't sound appealing at first, but when it comes to procrastination, one of the most effective strategies can be to embrace short-term discomfort. You don't need me to tell you that uncomfortable feelings only get worse the longer we delay the task. Instead of running away from these uncomfortable feelings, face them head-on and take action anyway. This is what I mean by embracing the suck: intentionally decide to lean into the dread, worry and resentment that you have to do it in the first place. Commit to feeling it, knowing that in doing so you're lessening the amount of time that you'll experience these feelings. With practice, this can become a powerful tool in your anti-procrastination toolkit. It will help you build emotional resilience and learn to navigate through discomfort, rather than trying to avoid it.

Reason with yourself

While I do think it's a good idea to do things that are fun and enjoyable, I'm not about to try and convince you that you should love every task in your life, because that just isn't going to happen. However, it's worth asking yourself if you actually want to do something and, whether you do or you don't, why? Asking this will either highlight your reason for doing it and provide some motivation for getting on with it or it will help uncover what the hold-up is. For instance, if I could avoid ever having to clean a toilet again, I would, but I can find plenty of reasons why cleaning toilets on a regular basis is a really good idea and I do it.

Spend a minute writing down all the reasons why doing this *now* is the best idea:

- Once I do it, it will be done
- I won't have to keep feeling this way
- It won't be hanging over me
- It won't occupy my brain for the rest of the day/week/year
- I will feel proud of myself
- I will be able to focus on the things I'd rather be doing
- I won't blame and shame myself
- I won't have to deal with forgetting about it (again)
- The timeline won't be delayed
- Doing this will allow others to move forwards with their work
- I can get back to doing my thing.

Set clear deadlines

I know it's an obvious one, but it can get missed and when it does Parkinson's Law can come into play. Parkinson's Law states that work expands to fill the time available for its completion. This means that if you give yourself a week to complete a two-hour task, then (psychologically speaking) the task will increase in complexity and become more daunting to fill that week. It may not even fill the extra time with more work, but just stress and tension about having to get it done.

In the context of procrastination, Parkinson's Law suggests that by setting shorter deadlines, the perceived complexity of the task reduces, making it easier to get started. Conversely, if you allow yourself a lot of time to complete a task, you're more likely to procrastinate, because the task seems more complex and daunting than it really is. Constraining the amount of time you allow yourself to spend on a task can make you more efficient and productive (as long the deadline is reasonable and doesn't lead to panic).

Small steps

Overcoming procrastination isn't about making giant leaps, it's about taking small, consistent steps forward. Every step, no matter how small, brings you closer to your goal of getting it done, so one of the most effective strategies for overcoming procrastination is to focus on taking one small step forward. This approach is based on the understanding that the hardest part of any task is often just getting started. Once we take that first step, it's easier to build and maintain momentum.

The beauty of this approach is that it reduces the mental and emotional resistance associated with the task. It's much easier to convince ourselves to do something small than something big. And once we take that first step, we often find that it's not as bad as we thought it would be. We start to build momentum and, before we know it, we're making progress on the task. For instance, if you need to send someone an email using this technique, you would open your email account and then focus on the next step – pulling up a blank email – then the next one, typing 'Hi' followed by their name. What's one sentence you want to say in the email? Type that. Is there something else that you want to add? Type that. This might sound excruciating, after all, it's 'just' an email, but as someone who goes to great lengths to avoid emails, I can tell you that this really works for my brain and it just might for yours, too.

This strategy works so well, because it shifts your focus from the outcome to the process. Instead of worrying about completing the task perfectly or how someone will respond, you focus on the act of doing. This reduces the fear and anxiety associated with the task, making it easier to get started. Remember, all you need is that first bit of momentum, so start with the bare minimum. This might be something as simple as writing the first sentence of a report, doing the first five minutes of a workout or sorting through the first pile of clutter in a room. You'll find that once you've started, you're more inclined to keep going.

Dopamine stacking

Procrastination occurs when we perceive a task is overwhelming, boring or lacking immediate rewards. Our brains crave instant gratification and when a task doesn't offer an immediate dopamine boost, we're more inclined to put it off.

Dopamine is a neurotransmitter that plays a crucial role in the brain's reward and pleasure centres, and it's associated with feelings of motivation, pleasure and reinforcement. When we engage in activities that provide a sense of reward or pleasure, such as accomplishing a task, receiving praise or experiencing small wins, the brain releases dopamine. This release of dopamine reinforces the behaviour and motivates us to continue engaging in similar activities.

Dopamine stacking refers to the practice of deliberately structuring tasks or activities in a way that allows for the accumulation of small, enjoyable rewards, successes and celebrations. For example, as I write this book, I'm actively choosing to celebrate each completed paragraph, section and chapter. By taking a moment to acknowledge my efforts and feel the satisfaction of what I've achieved, I continue to build the momentum that ultimately leads to a completed book. By breaking down larger tasks into smaller, more manageable steps and incorporating pleasurable elements into each step, we can create a sense of accomplishment and motivation to continue, making it more enticing and rewarding.

Temptation bundling

A concept developed by Katherine Milkman, a professor at the University of Pennsylvania's Wharton School, the idea behind temptation bundling is that you link a task that you should do, but are avoiding or procrastinating on, with a task that you love to do. By bundling these tasks together, you can make the less enjoyable task more appealing and reduce the likelihood of procrastination.

For example, if you love watching your favourite TV show, but know you want to be exercising more, you could bundle these tasks together. You only allow yourself to watch the show while you're on the treadmill or doing a workout at home. That way, you're more likely to look forward to exercising, because it's associated with something you enjoy.

In a research study conducted by Milkman, participants who had access to tempting audio novels only at the gym made 51 per cent more gym visits than those in the control group, promoting the desired positive behaviour change. You can even buy remote control rings that allow you to scroll hands-free on TikTok while on the treadmill!

However, although temptation bundling can be an effective technique, that doesn't mean it will work for everyone or for every type of job, especially if it's not practically possible to bundle two activities together. The two tasks need to be done concurrently and when the enjoyable task is something that can be used as a reward, but not to the point where the temptation task distracts from, or reduces the effectiveness of, the task you're trying to complete.

Ante up

This technique is most productive in situations that are about long-term goals and behaviours. It works by bringing the consequences of not doing something forward in time. If a deadline or the consequences of not completing a task seem far off in the future, you may feel less urgency about acting now. This is often referred to as temporal discounting, where we value immediate rewards more than future rewards.

In terms of procrastination, this might mean choosing to watch a movie now (immediate reward) rather than studying for an exam that's a week away (future reward). As the deadline gets closer, the future consequences become more immediate and the urgency to act increases. This is why people often end up cramming for exams or rushing to meet deadlines at the last minute.

Time inconsistency (also known as temporal inconsistency) is a concept in behavioural economics that describes the tendency of people to make different choices based on the timing of the decision. This concept is closely related to procrastination and essentially means that we value immediate rewards more than future rewards. This is known as hyperbolic discounting: when a reward is far off in the future, we tend to discount its value.

However, as the reward (or deadline) gets closer, its perceived value increases. This can lead to inconsistent decisions over time. For example, someone might decide today that they will start a new exercise programme next Monday (why must we always start these things on Mondays?!), valuing the future benefit of improved physical and mental health. But, when Monday rolls around and it's time to do it, the immediate pleasure of sitting around watching Netflix is possibly going to outweigh the future benefit of exercising, leading them to delay taking action.

Again, this isn't a you thing. As humans, we are prone to delaying tasks that have future benefits, but require immediate effort, in favour of activities that provide immediate pleasure or relief. But as the deadline for the task gets closer, the immediate negative consequences of not doing the task (a bad grade, a missed deadline) become more tangible and you're more likely to finally take action. Ways that you can up the ante include:

- Creating artificial deadlines or milestones along the way: Large tasks and long-term goals can feel overwhelming, which can lead to procrastination. Breaking them down into smaller, manageable tasks can make it easier to get started, so create artificial deadlines or milestones that break down the task into smaller, more immediate goals. This can help to reduce the time discrepancy and make the future consequences feel more immediate, providing a greater sense of urgency to act now. For instance, rather than have the goal of writing an entire book, I have a daily word count that I task myself with hitting no matter what.
- Using accountability partners: Share your goals and deadlines with a friend, colleague, or mentor. Knowing that someone else is aware of your commitments – or even joining you in them – can provide an extra push to get started.
- Implementing immediate consequences: Create a system where there are real consequences if you don't complete a task. This can be anything from paying a friend £5 every time a deadline is missed to a social penalty, such as not doing something you've been looking forward to (just be mindful this doesn't stray into punishment and self-flagellation). I don't let myself send text messages to my friends until I've hit my word count for the day.

- Using reward systems: On the flip side, rewarding yourself for completing tasks can also be a powerful motivator. This could be a small treat, a break to do something you enjoy or a larger reward for completing a big project. (In case you were wondering, my reward for handing the manuscript for this book in is having a horse-riding lesson every day for a week.)
- Visualising the negative outcomes: Spend some time thinking about the negative consequences of not completing the task. For example, you might visualise the negative consequences of not studying for the exam, such as failing the course or not getting the grade you want, the disappointment of missing an opportunity or the negative impact on your reputation.

Each step you take, no matter how uncomfortable, brings you closer to where you want to be. And in doing so, we not only achieve our goals, but also make life easier for our future selves. Above all, remember it's always how you respond to a situation that matters.

Chapter 3

Defensiveness

Defensiveness is that prickly, knee-jerk reaction that pops up when we feel attacked, criticised or, heaven forbid, when someone suggests we might be wrong about something. Defensiveness, in all its glory, is a universal human behaviour. It's like that uninvited guest who shows up at every party, eats all the snacks and manages to rub everyone up the wrong way. We've all been there, haven't we? One minute we're having a perfectly pleasant conversation and the next we're puffing up like an offended porcupine, ready to launch our quills at anyone who dares to challenge us.

But defensiveness isn't inherently bad. It's a natural response designed to protect us from perceived threats. It's part of our survival mechanism, deeply rooted in our biology and psychology. When our beliefs, values or self-image are threatened, our brain goes into defence mode, activating our SRS and preparing us to fight, flee or freeze.

The problem arises when our defensiveness gets in the way of effective communication, hinders personal and professional growth, and damages our relationships. When we're constantly on guard, ready to defend ourselves at a moment's notice, we close ourselves off to connection and intimacy with others, new ideas, constructive criticism and opportunities for growth. We become like a castle with its drawbridge permanently up, safe and secure, but also isolated and stagnant.

So, how do we lower our drawbridge without leaving ourselves vulnerable to attack? How do we navigate the fine line between self-protection and self-sabotage? That's what we're going to explore in this chapter, but before we dive in, let's take a moment to appreciate the irony of this situation.

Here we are, about to delve into a chapter on defensiveness, and I bet there's a part of you that's already feeling a bit defensive. 'I'm not defensive,' you might be thinking. 'I'm just passionate. And right. Mostly right.' And that, my friend, is the beauty of defensiveness. It's so ingrained in our behaviour that often we don't even realise we're doing it. But don't worry, we're in this together. So, let's take a deep breath, check our porcupine quills at the door and dive in, shall we?

The Nervous System Shield

Defensiveness, at its core, is a protective mechanism. It's your way of saying, 'Hey, I feel threatened here and I need to protect myself.' It's a reaction to perceived criticism, judgement or attack, and it often manifests as a counterattack or withdrawal. You know the drill: someone points out a mistake you made and, before you know it, you're either launching into a passionate monologue about why you're not wrong or you're retreating into icy silence.

When faced with a perceived threat, your instinctual response kicks in, triggering defensiveness as a means of self-preservation. At the core of defensiveness lies your body's SRS, governed by the autonomic nervous system. This system acts as our personal security system, primed to react when danger is perceived, whether it's a physical threat or an attack on our self-esteem. The familiar fight, flight or freeze responses come into play, each with its own unique characteristics.

Fight and flight are defensive strategies that diverge in their actions and intentions. The fight response involves moving *towards* the perceived threat, embodying a sense of power, control and even dominance. It's what I describe as 'posturing up'; making ourselves bigger to assert our presence and ward off potential harm. Flight, on the other hand, prompts us to move *away* from the threat, seeking safety by putting distance between ourselves and the source of danger.

While fight and flight are fairly overt in their manifestations, the freeze response operates in a more subtle manner. From an external perspective, it may appear as if nothing is happening, but internally there is a whirlwind of activity. The freeze response involves a heightened state of internal activation, where our body and mind prepare for potential threats without making any obvious external movements. It's as if time momentarily stands still as our system assesses the situation and determines the best course of action.

Understanding these different responses sheds light on the multifaceted nature of defensiveness. It reveals how our survival instincts influence our reactions, shaping our behaviours in the face of perceived threats.

Defensiveness is a complex physiological response, deeply ingrained in our biology and psychology – a testament to your body's incredible capacity to protect you from harm. But, as we'll explore in the next sections, it's also something that we can learn to manage and regulate, for the sake of our personal growth and our relationships.

Highway to the Danger Zone

In the film, *Top Gun: Maverick*, actor Tom Cruise reprises his role as naval aviator Pete 'Maverick' Mitchell. His role is to train a group of elite Top Gun graduates to complete a specialist mission that has very little chance of success. Their objective is to destroy a uranium enrichment plant in a rogue state, flying their fighter jets fast and low through a deep valley to avoid detection by a whole load of anti-aircraft missiles perched on the surrounding mountains.

In one scene, we see what happens when the missiles detect an aircraft, instantly swivelling to face the threat and launch a missile at Mach 4 speeds. It's a swift, automatic response to a perceived threat. And it's a perfect metaphor for defensiveness. When we feel threatened – whether it's a criticism from a partner, a negative comment from a colleague or a dismissive gesture from a friend – our internal missile system springs into action.

There are times when it's necessary and helpful for your missile defence system to be activated and there are times when it's over-reactive. Imagine if, in *Top Gun*, the missile system detects movement, but it's not a fighter jet, it's a kitten. No sense in going to the trouble of launching surface-to-air missiles for a kitten, is there? Not every perceived threat warrants a missile launch. Doing so would be an overreaction, and it can cause unnecessary conflict and strain in our relationships.

So, how do we prevent these unnecessary missile launches? How do we ensure that our defensiveness doesn't get in the way of open, honest communication? The key is to recognise when your missile system is being over-reactive; to pause and assess the situation before you launch your counterattack; to ask yourself whether that's a fighter jet coming at you or a kitten. Easier said than done, I know. This requires self-awareness, mindfulness and emotional regulation. It requires us to tune into our bodies, to recognise the early signs of defensiveness and, when appropriate, soothe our nervous system before we react. It also requires us to practise open, assertive communication; to express our feelings and needs in a respectful, constructive way, without resorting to defensiveness.

Survival Mode Versus Learning Mode

Your brain operates in two modes: survival mode and learning mode. In survival mode, your SRS is activated and fear-based thinking takes over. This is when your survival brain kicks in, hyperfocusing on the perceived threat, demonstrating a low tolerance of ambiguity and thinking in black and white terms. In this mode, we are fearful of making mistakes and just concerned with getting through it. Survival mode, as the name implies, is all about safety and survival, and is therefore more reactionary. This mode is perfect when there's an actual threat to deal with, but perhaps less helpful when someone's simply asking if they can help you with a task.

In the absence of a perceived threat, learning mode is brought online. In this mode, we are open to receiving new information, curious, interested and able to learn. We can handle ambiguity and are less afraid of making mistakes. In learning mode, the brain is goal-oriented and approaches problem-solving creatively; it is solution-focused.

It's easy to assume that the learning brain is somehow better than the survival brain, but that's not the case. They each have their own unique skill sets, we just want the right brain for the right job, because although the ability to jump into fight or flight can be lifesaving, there are times when this defence mechanism isn't needed, but your body will be convinced that it is and you'll respond as though you're being attacked when you aren't.

A few years ago, I had a huge realisation about my romantic relationship. My historic tendency has been to respond to anything that felt even mildly confrontational by immediately jumping to, 'Why am I even with him? I should leave and get out of this situation.' Now while there have been relationships when that was a wise move, I have also experienced this response in my current loving relationship of 10 years, which I have absolutely no desire to leave, all because my survival brain was activated and a very old operating system kicked in, complete with flashing red lights designed to convince me that there was a threat I needed to get away from. Thankfully, there was no actual threat, just my loving partner wanting to talk about something important in a very non-threatening way, but that didn't stop my SRS from running its threat detection programme.

Black and White Thinking

Black and white thinking is the tendency to see things in extremes and it prevents you from seeing the middle ground. It's a binary pattern of thinking that psychologists refer to as a cognitive distortion, because it blocks you from seeing life for what it is – uncertain, nuanced and forever changing. Black and white thinking (aka splitting) results in seeing things as wrong or right, good or bad, or that there are only two possible options.

Cognitive distortions such as this are associated with ADHD, autism, depression, borderline personality disorder (BPD) and narcissistic personality disorder (NPD), but it's worth remembering that black and white thinking is something *all humans* do from time to time, especially when your survival brain is running the show. Think about a time when you've felt stressed and overwhelmed, and the pressure of the situation has meant your survival brain jumped into action and you couldn't think clearly or creatively. My bet is that in times like that it's hard to see all the options available to you, because your brain goes into this or that mode – *'There are only two options and you'd better pick the right one or we're doomed'* – and it takes someone else to say, 'But what about doing it like this instead?' for you to realise that there are other options that include a great solution.

When your stress response system has been activated like this, your thinking brain isn't available and it's extraordinarily hard to find the shades of grey. Even when someone is using their thinking brain to provide a perfect solution, you might be unable to hear and accept it until your stress response system has been disarmed. In fact, you may even perceive them as a threat for coming up with a solution when you couldn't.

Heavy Load

Some days it feels like you can handle things, effortlessly dealing with whatever comes your way – *I got this, no problem* – but on other days even the smallest things can feel like too much and push you over the edge. You end up snapping, hiding in a bathroom or descending into a doom spiral while sitting at your desk. Let me explain why...

Your SRS has a threshold – a tipping point where your fight, flight or freeze responses are activated. Ideally, when these responses kick in, you take appropriate action to deal with the perceived threat or recognise that the response is unnecessary. In either case, a state of resolution is reached and you return to a regulated state. But life isn't always perfect and this ideal scenario doesn't always play out, especially when you're not fully aware of how your nervous system functions and how to work with it.

Instead, what often happens is that you get stuck in a stress response. As you go through your day, each stress response adds to the previous ones, accumulating like weights in a backpack. Without sufficient resolution and recovery, the seemingly insignificant things become magnified. That's when you find yourself losing it, because there's a sock on the floor that shouldn't be there – the same sock that was there this morning and didn't bother you at all because your stress response system was at its baseline rather than its threshold.

Dysregulation of your SRS can cause an initial over-responsiveness and if this becomes the norm then a hypersensitivity can develop, intensifying the cues from your internal and external environment, and decreasing your capacity to handle common challenges, such as things not going to plan and criticism from others. This can lead to hypervigilance and exaggerated responses that aren't necessary and may even be inaccurate, so even though your SRS is trying to keep you alive, it needs reminding that someone asking you a question doesn't warrant the body equivalent of an armoured response team.

If stress continues and isn't addressed, your SRS gradually becomes less responsive and, while a reduction in stress sensitivity may sound great and in some ways is probably quite a wise way of your SRS protecting you, it also means you're less likely to respond to internal and external situations that it would be beneficial for you to respond to. While there are times in which being more responsive or less responsive is valuable in the moment, the trouble comes when this becomes established as your SRS's baseline way of operating.

The first step in managing defensiveness is to notice and name your stress responses. By acknowledging the physical sensations, and patterns of tension and relaxation in your body, you can become more attuned to the early signs of stress and defensiveness. This heightened awareness allows you to question the accuracy and relevance of the information your body is providing. While your experiences are valid, the information your body is giving you may be rooted in past experiences that are not necessarily useful in the present moment.

Managing defensiveness is not about eliminating it entirely, as it serves a protective function. Rather, it's about recognising its presence and learning to navigate it more effectively. By cultivating body awareness and consciously questioning the validity of your stress responses, you can gain greater control over your reactions. This dance with defensiveness becomes an opportunity for self-reflection and growth, allowing you to respond to stress with greater resilience and emotional intelligence.

Interoception and Emotional Regulation

Let's dive into the deep end of the pool for a moment and talk about the SRS, interoception and emotional regulation. Sounds like a mouthful, but bear with me, because understanding these concepts can give us valuable insights into our defensiveness.

Interoception is our ability to sense what's happening inside our bodies. It's like our body's internal GPS, guiding us towards our emotional and physical needs. When we're in tune with our interoceptive signals, we can recognise the early signs of stress and take steps to manage it effectively (see pages 130–4 for more on interoception).

The SRS, on the other hand, is our body's built-in alarm system. It prepares us to respond to threats and maintain our equilibrium. It involves several subsystems, each with its own unique response to stress. When the SRS is dysregulated – due to chronic stress, for example – it can lead to hyperresponsivity (overreacting to stress) or hyporesponsivity (underreacting to stress). Both can affect our relationship with our bodies and emotions, leading to either hypervigilance or decreased responsiveness.

Ongoing stress can affect our interoceptive awareness by altering the intensity of our internal cues and how we perceive and interpret them. This means that stress can influence multiple levels of our interoceptive process, from the strength of our internal signals to our ability to tolerate and interpret these signals.

Stress responses are adaptive, helping us cope with challenging environments, but problems arise when these responses remain 'set', even when the environment changes. This can occur in two distinct ways: when the SRS is stuck on high or stuck on low.

When the SRS is stuck on high, it's like having a smoke alarm that never stops blaring. Even in situations where there is no real danger, your body continues to react as if it's under imminent threat. This heightened state of arousal can leave you feeling on edge, overwhelmed and constantly on guard.

Everyday stressors that would typically be manageable become amplified, leading to increased tension, irritability and difficulty in finding a sense of calm. If you're hypersensitive to stress, you might become overly defensive, reacting strongly to minor criticisms or challenges. It's as if your nervous system has cranked up the volume on the stress response dial, causing the slightest trigger to unleash a cascade of physiological and emotional reactions.

When the SRS is stuck on low, it's like having a faulty smoke alarm that never goes off, even when it needs to. Your body's stress response becomes dampened and unresponsive, resulting in an overall blunted reactivity. While this might sound appealing at first, because it diminishes the intensity of the stress, it also dampens your ability to engage with, and respond effectively to, both internal and external challenges.

You may find yourself feeling detached, numb and disengaged from the world around you. It becomes difficult to muster the necessary energy and motivation to tackle tasks or deal with potential stressors. In this state, your stress response system has turned down the volume so low that it struggles to recognise and appropriately respond to cues that require activation and engagement, including when you need to be defensive! Just as a pendulum swings from one extreme to another, finding equilibrium requires finding the sweet spot in the middle.

Client Story

Emily, a 42-year-old working mother of three and client of mine, found herself perpetually swinging between feeling on edge and feeling completely numb. At one point, Emily's SRS never seemed to stop blaring. She was juggling her demanding job, her children's needs and the household chores. Even minor challenges, like misplaced keys or a short delay in traffic, sent her into a spiral of anxiety. She became hypersensitive, overreacting to minor criticisms and offers of help from her spouse, and snapping at her children over trivial matters. It felt like the volume on her stress response was turned up to the max and she was constantly on guard.

After a period of feeling stressed and on edge, she became overwhelmed, disengaged and numb to the world around her. She withdrew, and struggled to recognise and respond to cues that required engagement, including defending herself when necessary, like when her colleague went on a tirade against her in a team meeting. Through coaching, Emily began the process of locating the sweet spot between these two extremes. She learned to recognise when her SRS was either too high or too low, and learned to find the middle ground.

Window of Tolerance

In the realm of psychology and trauma therapy, there's a concept known as the 'window of tolerance'. This term, coined by professor of psychiatry, Dr Dan Siegel, refers to the zone of arousal in which a person can function most effectively. When we're within our window of tolerance, we're able to effectively manage and respond to the daily ups and downs of life. We can think clearly, make rational decisions and process what's going on within us and around us.

In this optimal zone, we can play, learn and be in relationships with ourselves and others. We are calm and alert, aware of the options available to us. When you are within the window of tolerance, your SRS will be activated, but you're able to experience the activation and move through it. Imagine you're about to cross a road and, just as you step off the pavement, a car you didn't notice turns the corner, causing you to swiftly move backwards, out of harm's way. Your SRS would kick into gear with a cascade of events that happen before your brain's visual centres have had a chance to process what you've seen. Adrenaline is released, your heart rate and breathing accelerate, and your muscles respond by getting you to move out of the way. It is a shock, but it's part and parcel of living among cars and you've probably experienced it before, so unless it was a near miss, you'll operate within your window of tolerance and your SRS soon settles down again.

This see-saw of activation and deactivation allows you to meet the challenges of daily life, and there are fluctuations in mood and energy levels too, but while you're within the window of tolerance, you're able to both soothe and stimulate yourself sufficiently, and adjust to what happens, becoming neither too reactive nor too withdrawn in response to the circumstances. Wonderful! But we also need to talk about what happens when you move outside your window of tolerance – when you can't calm down or you start to shut down altogether.

When you move beyond your window of tolerance into a state of *hyper*arousal, you'll experience:

- Fight/flight activation
- Impaired judgement
- Things feeling like they're too much
- Inability to calm down
- Emotional reactivity
- Impulsivity
- Anger
- Aggression
- Defensiveness
- Agitation
- Distress
- Panic
- Tension
- Hypervigilance
- Rigid thinking
- Rumination.

*Hypo*arousal has a different set of qualities to it:

- Freeze response
- Withdrawal
- Feeling too little
- An absence of sensations
- Feeling numb or empty
- Loneliness
- A sense of hopelessness
- Passivity
- Inability to think or respond
- Shutting down
- Low energy and mood
- Feeling flat or depressed
- Feeling disconnected
- Dissociation.

Although your experience of them probably feels awful, neither hyperarousal nor hypoarousal are bad per se; they are merely mechanisms that have evolved to protect us from danger and distress.

When you operate outside your window of tolerance, your ability to focus, see the big picture, figure out the problem and come up with a solution all go out the window with you, and so does your willpower. When you're outside your window of tolerance, you're susceptible to feeling overwhelmed, and an inability to think clearly and creatively can prevent you from making decisions effectively – your capacity and resilience are reduced. My experience of being in this situation is that I can't see the blindingly obvious solution to something and it takes someone else saying, 'What about this?' for me to realise there is an easy way to solve things.

The window of tolerance doesn't have set measurements, so it will vary from one person to another. Everyone's window of tolerance is different. For some it might be wide, allowing them to handle a high level of stress or stimulation without becoming overwhelmed. For others it might be narrow, meaning they become stressed and overwhelmed more easily.

It will also fluctuate for an individual – your capacity to handle life's challenges will be affected by physical and mental health, pain, emotional state, lack of sleep, feeling hungry, fluctuating hormone levels during the menstrual cycle and perimenopause transition, and past experiences with stress or trauma. For instance, if we're already feeling stressed, our window of tolerance may shrink, making us more prone to defensiveness or other reactive behaviours.

Understanding your window of tolerance can be incredibly helpful in managing defensiveness. If we know that our window of tolerance is narrow, we can take steps to expand it, such as practising stress management techniques, improving our self-care routines, or seeking support from a therapist or coach. We can also learn to recognise when we're approaching the edges of our window of tolerance and take steps to soothe our nervous system before we become overwhelmed.

We all have different baselines and thresholds. Those who've experienced neglect, abuse, trauma and adverse childhood experiences (ACEs – see pages 49–50) are more likely to struggle to regulate themselves and experience the co-regulation that comes from receiving the nurturing connection of another person, resulting in a narrower window of tolerance. This, in turn, causes an individual to be quicker to detect real or perceived threats, causing further activation of the SRS and the possibility of them living in a chronically activated state.

Those with early experiences of trauma, and those who grew up in environments that were emotionally and/or physically unsafe, attempt to keep themselves safer by constantly scanning their surroundings and assessing for potential threats – what is known as hypervigilance.

In the 'right' environment, all humans are capable of hypervigilance, because it's what allows us to be highly sensitive to our surroundings. It's an ability that's incredibly useful if you hear an unusual noise in your home or if you're in a setting where someone could try to steal your belongings, but it can become all-consuming.

Client Story

My client Bashak was experiencing stress, loneliness and anxiety, always thinking that the world would burst into flames. She feared situations like going bankrupt and felt hijacked by stress responses. On top of that, she felt like she was the only one having these issues.

In learning about her stress responses, Bashak realised that she'd spent most of her life in fight/flight mode and she identified this as the main cause of her autoimmunity health issues: 'A big part of it was the environment I grew up in. It really wasn't surprising that I was under high stress all the time, but I didn't realise it at the time, because, in a country where collective traumas are occurring every day, you don't trust anything or anyone – that's the norm.

'I made so many of my decisions from fear. Decision-making was freaking scary before I started working with Maisie, but now it's one of my best things, because it gives me clarity. New helpful thoughts have been easier to cultivate with the help of good coaches and a supportive community. A big part of it is also because I'm a social animal who needs other humans! I'm more grounded, loving and more of an individual. I can express my needs and wishes better, I don't take things personally and I can set boundaries.'

Adverse Childhood Experiences

In 1995, a groundbreaking study was conducted by the Centers for Disease Control (CDC) and Kaiser Permanente healthcare organisation in California. The study looked at how children's sense of safety, stability and bonding might be undermined by the impact of adverse childhood experiences (ACEs – potentially traumatic events that occur in childhood, defined as from birth to age 17), specifically:

- Physical or emotional abuse
- Neglect
- Household dysfunction
- Caregiver mental illness
- Substance use in a child's environment
- Instability due to parental separation or household members being in prison
- Having a family member attempt or die by suicide
- Witnessing violence in the home or community.

The researchers found that adverse childhood experiences (ACEs) were common, with 61 per cent of the US population having experienced at least one ACE and 16 per cent having experienced four or more. In a 2014 UK study on ACEs, 47 per cent of people had experienced at least one ACE, with 9 per cent of the population experiencing four or more.

There is a powerful and persistent relationship between the number of ACEs experienced and poor outcomes later in life; the greater the number of ACEs, the greater the chance of developing heart disease, diabetes, depression, substance abuse, smoking and early death. ACEs can negatively impact education and academic achievement, job opportunities, time out of employment and earning potential as well.

The US researchers found that women and several racial/ethnic groups are at greater risk of experiencing four or more ACEs and noted the impact of the social determinants of health, such as living in under-resourced or racially segregated neighbourhoods, frequently moving or experiencing food insecurity (according to a Food Foundation report, in September 2022, 25 per cent of children were experiencing this in the UK).

ACEs can leave an enduring imprint on the SRS, shaping how an individual responds to stress throughout their life. The early years are a critical period in which the foundations of the SRS are established. Exposure to ACEs during this sensitive time can disrupt its normal development, leading to lasting changes.

At the heart of this alteration is the concept of stress sensitisation. Early life stress can create a lower threshold for stress reactivity, making the system more easily triggered by subsequent stressors. This heightened sensitivity isn't merely a temporary state; it can become a chronic condition that persists into adulthood, influencing both mental and physical health. The stress sensitisation theory highlights how early adversity can change the biological 'set point' of the stress response, causing it to activate more readily and with more intensity.

Stress in childhood doesn't simply dissipate; it can multiply and extend into various aspects of adult life. Exposure to ACEs can increase the risk of encountering additional adversities, creating a cascading effect. Childhood adversity might lead to secondary stressors that act together with, or replace, the initial event, leading to compounded health consequences.

The interplay between early life stress, socioeconomic factors and later life adversity adds another layer of complexity to how ACEs influence the stress response. An individual's race, ethnicity (or rather other people's response to their race and ethnicity), availability of material resources and social status can intersect with early life stress to shape a unique stress response profile.

Understanding the profound connection between ACEs and the stress response system is essential, as recognising that early life experiences may be at the core of an individual's stress reactivity helps to create more nuanced and targeted interventions. By addressing both the historical roots and present manifestations of stress, therapy and support can be tailored to meet the unique needs of those who have experienced ACEs, promoting understanding, resilience and recovery.

A lot of my work involves helping clients to notice what causes them to slip outside their window of tolerance; to become aware of when they're moving out of their optimal zone; and to find ways of collaborating with their SRS so that they're able to tend to themselves in the moment and create a felt sense of safety within themselves. Once that foundation has been established, then we're able to focus on expanding their capacity, so that they can respond to greater challenges, whatever that looks like for them, whether it's receiving praise, initiating a difficult conversation or experiencing discomfort in some way.

Client Story

This is what my client Naomi says about her challenges: 'I wanted to create the safety in myself again; to fully feel and express freely; to overcome fear of failure, shame and judgement; and to build on the work I've done in changing past beliefs and growing my self-esteem, boundaries, assertion and worth. Self-worth and self-love weren't always modelled for me growing up. I felt very unsafe and unlovable. My mother also kept small and played safe, and avoided failure, so that's what was modelled to me.

'Bit by bit I'm trusting that things can be different, and to feel safe within myself again and who I am. I'm challenging unhelpful or dubious thoughts in the moment. I love that I'm able to work with my nervous system and take care of myself through movement, breath and meditation. I'm also learning it's okay to ask for help.'

Many of my clients describe having a different window of tolerance when they're approaching ovulation compared to the days when they're approaching their period. In the run-up to ovulation, hormone levels of oestrogen and testosterone are peaking, all with the aim of getting you to go out, find a mate and have sex while you're in the fertile window (the phase of the menstrual cycle in which conception is possible). As such, these hormones often result in you feeling more confident, social and chatty, as well as being associated with an increase in risk-taking and sexual desire.

Conversely, in the second half of the cycle, hormone levels are there to support a possible pregnancy. The ebb and flow of hormones through the menstrual cycle impacts mood, energy and behaviour.

Client Story

My client Harriet describes her experience like this: 'Around ovulation I feel like I can take on the world and problems can even feel fun to solve, but a week or so later the same issue feels completely different, and I get overwhelmed and stressed about things instead. My tolerance level varies with my cycle, but now that I'm aware of it, I can plan around it... I slow down and am gentler with myself in the days before my period starts.'

The Great Wall of Defensiveness

When you're feeling dysregulated, your body might be in a state of hyperarousal or hypoarousal or you may be bouncing between the two. You can probably think of someone in your life who's quick to get angry and defensive, and someone else who's more likely to defend themselves by withdrawing. Many of my clients will alternate between these dysregulated states. For example, they will go through an intense period of work, with long days, insufficient breaks, late nights, poor sleep, getting through the day on caffeine, sugar and carbs, and with little to no time for rest and rejuvenation, but this will typically be followed by a post-deadline crash of some kind, where they're unable to get out of bed or off the sofa until they've soothed their nervous system sufficiently.

Living in a state of stress for days, weeks, months or years adds up. Without sufficient resolution and recovery to bring you back to your baseline, stress levels – and defensive behaviour – creep up and up, and before you know it, you're hanging out at your threshold most or all of the time. A common scenario that I've observed in myself and my clients is the pressure of looming deadlines; as the intensity of a project increases and more is required of you, your regular working hours and meals are ditched, and late nights, caffeine and takeaways are embraced.

Without awareness and intervention (because it *is* possible to do things differently), you find yourself bracing yourself and adopting an 'I just need to get through this' mentality, because you're existing all the way up at your threshold. A bit of sleep, a nutritious meal, spending time outside or stroking a pet might provide enough regulation to create some distance from your threshold, but, overall, it won't be enough to bring you back down to your baseline. Again, there's nothing wrong with doing this occasionally, but we don't want it to become the norm.

Sometimes when I explain this to people, they assume that I'm telling them that they have to make a choice between getting their work done or taking care of themselves, and there are times when that will be the case – typically when someone is so burnt out that their system needs a reset or when they're doing a super-human amount of work that simply isn't do-able or sustainable. Most of the time, though, that's not what we're talking about and my belief is that it is possible to get your work done and meet deadlines while also taking care of yourself. These two things do not have to be in opposition to each other, but of course we've been socialised to believe that it's one or the other.

Listen, I want you to get your shit done, I'm all for it, I just don't want you wrecking yourself in the process. But it's not just that, there are other concerning consequences, such as deepening the belief that this is the only way to do life. Remember that everything you do is either deepening neural grooves or creating new pathways, and this is why it's so valuable to find other ways of getting things done, methods that bring out the best in you without costing you and leaving you stressed, burnt out and no good to anyone.

Chronic stress can dial up your defensiveness. If you're constantly under stress, your body hangs out in a heightened state of arousal, ready to respond to perceived threats, making you more reactive and prone to defensiveness, and less able to effectively manage your emotions. Chronic stress can lead to a variety of physical and mental health problems, including anxiety, depression, heart disease and a weakened immune system. It can also shrink our window of tolerance, making us more susceptible to overwhelm and less able to cope with additional stressors.

Overactivation of the stress response system can lead to chronic stress, which in turn can have a host of negative effects on our physical and mental health. It can also fuel defensiveness, as we find ourselves constantly on guard, ready to fight off perceived threats. When we're under chronic stress, our bodies are constantly on high alert, ready to launch into a stress response at the slightest sign of threat. This can make us more likely to perceive others' words or actions as threats, triggering our defensiveness. It can also make it harder for us to think clearly, communicate effectively and respond to feedback in a constructive way.

A Double-edged Sword

Defensiveness, while often seen as a barrier to effective communication and personal growth, is an asset in certain professions. Some people make entire careers out of defending themselves or their clients.

In the world of business, defensiveness can be a valuable strategy. Business leaders often need to defend their decisions, their teams and their companies against criticism and competition. A certain level of defensiveness can be protective, helping them to stand their ground, assert their vision and navigate the cutthroat world of corporate politics.

Similarly, in the legal profession, lawyers are tasked with defending their clients' interests and this can require a certain level of defensiveness – challenging opposing arguments, questioning evidence and pushing back against unfavourable interpretations of the law. In this context, defensiveness is not just useful, it's essential.

However, while defensiveness can be an asset in these contexts, it can also have its downsides, particularly when it comes to stress. Being constantly on the defensive can be exhausting. It can keep your stress response system in a state of high alert, leading to chronic stress, and all the physical and mental health problems that come with it, including:

- Cardiovascular issues: Chronic stress has been linked to heart problems such as high blood pressure, heart disease and even heart attacks.
- Digestive problems: Stress can disrupt the digestive system, inhibiting the body's ability to process food, causing discomfort and leading to long-term issues such as indigestion, acid reflux or irritable bowel syndrome (IBS).
- Immune system suppression: Chronic stress and the persistent production of stress hormones suppresses the immune system, hindering the body's ability to fight off diseases, leading to more frequent illnesses.
- Sleep disorders: I doubt you'll be surprised to hear that being in a constant state of alertness because of stress affects the body's ability to relax and fall asleep – if sleep disorders such as insomnia develop, they can, in turn, affect overall well-being, energy levels and cognitive function.
- Musculoskeletal pain: The physical tension caused by stress can lead to muscular aches, pains and strains, because chronic stress often results in tightened muscles, which, aside from causing discomfort, can contribute to conditions such as chronic back or neck pain.

- Metabolic changes: Stress can lead to unhealthy eating habits and weight fluctuations, resulting in metabolic issues that increase the risk of developing type 2 diabetes.
- Reproductive issues: Chronic stress can affect reproductive health by leading to disruptions in hormonal balances, which can result in menstrual irregularities and erectile dysfunction.

The defensiveness that serves us in the workplace doesn't always serve us in our personal lives. The same defensiveness that helps a lawyer win a case or a business leader to secure a deal can hinder open, honest communication with loved ones, making it difficult to hear feedback, acknowledge mistakes and accept personal responsibility.

Not Always the Bad Guy

Defensiveness gets a bad rap and for good reason – it can hinder communication, escalate conflicts, prevent us from hearing and taking on valuable feedback, and cause disconnection in relationships. But let's not forget that defensiveness also has its place. It's a natural response designed to protect us from harm, and there are situations where it's both appropriate and useful.

Microaggressions are subtle forms of discrimination that are directed towards individuals based on their race, ethnicity, gender, sexual orientation or other marginalised identities. Microaggressions are incredibly damaging, chipping away at a person's sense of self-worth and belonging over time. When it comes to microaggressions, defensiveness can serve as a protective mechanism, helping individuals to assert themselves and challenge discriminatory behaviour. The problem is that once someone does assert themselves, they are then likely to receive additional microaggressions. For example, if a white woman touches a Black woman's hair and is then told not to, there is a huge tendency for white women to respond by labelling Black women as aggressive and scary, or to state, 'I'm not racist, I've got friends who are Black', all of which are additional microaggressions.

Cultural bias is another area where defensiveness can play a crucial role. In a world where certain cultures and ways of life are privileged over others, defensiveness can help individuals to resist cultural erasure and assert the validity of their own experiences. For instance, consider the reaction of indigenous communities when their traditions or spiritual practices are appropriated or misrepresented in mainstream media. When a fashion brand uses sacred symbols as mere accessories, or when a festival-goer wears a traditional headdress as a costume, members of the indigenous community may respond defensively. This defensiveness is not about rejecting outside interest or being uncooperative; rather, it's a mechanism to protect the sanctity and authenticity of their cultural practices, to resist their culture being trivialised, and to assert the validity and depth of their own lived experiences.

Defensiveness can be a useful tool with gender bias. Our voices and experiences are often undervalued and dismissed, and defensiveness can help women to assert their boundaries, challenge sexist assumptions, and advocate for our rights and needs. Take, for instance, the context of a corporate meeting. Imagine a woman presenting a well-researched proposal, only to be interrupted or to have her ideas casually attributed to a male colleague later. In such a situation, her defensiveness can manifest as a firm, assertive response: 'I'd like to finish my point,' or 'To clarify, that was my proposal we're discussing.' By doing so, she's not just standing up for herself in the moment; she's challenging the gender bias that might assume her contributions are less valuable or noteworthy. This act of defensiveness becomes a tool to break the cycle of women's voices being overshadowed in professional settings.

In all these situations, defensiveness is not just about protecting the ego, it's about protecting one's dignity and rights in the face of systemic bias and discrimination, and defending oneself in a world that often seeks to silence and marginalise. However, for any of this to change, it requires those who are being discriminatory to stop being so defensive and actually listen and accept what they are being told.

Socialisation

From the moment we're born, our socialisation begins. Socialisation – the process through which we learn the norms, values and behaviours of our society – plays a significant role in shaping our defensiveness. From a young age we're taught how to respond to criticism, how to handle conflict and how to protect ourselves from perceived threats.

Girls are socialised into roles that require us to be nurturing, accommodating and selfless. One way or another, we're taught to put others' needs before our own, to be polite and to avoid conflict. This socialisation process can lead us to feel 'othered' and seen as wrong when we don't conform to these expectations. The pressure to conform can then lead to a heightened sense of defensiveness. After all, when you're constantly being criticised or judged for not fitting into a certain mould, it's natural to want to defend yourself. And there are certainly times when it's appropriate for us to be defensive, such as when we're facing discrimination.

Societal expectations and pressures can also contribute to defensiveness. We live in a society that values perfection, achievement and conformity. We're constantly bombarded with messages about how we should look, how we should behave and what we should achieve. This can create a pervasive sense of not being 'good enough', which can trigger defensiveness. But, as we've discussed, constant defensiveness can be exhausting and counterproductive. It can prevent us from hearing constructive criticism, learning from our mistakes and growing as individuals. It can also strain our relationships and create unnecessary conflict.

Regulating Resources

You already use regulating resources to soothe yourself because they are simply the things that you do – either on your own or with another – that enable you to come out of a stress response and into a regulated state. Regulating resources help to complete stress responses, support the nervous system and can be used to self-soothe. They help you to soften, relax and feel a sense of safety. They bring you back into feeling connected to yourself, others and the world around you.

What works for one person could very well be different from what works for another and it will vary depending on how you're feeling, too. Receiving a hug when you feel upset might be exactly what you need, but it might not work so well if you're in the fight stress response, because your missile system might need to be deactivated first.

When my son was a baby and we were trying to decorate our home, I spent hours and hours looking at paint charts while cuddling and feeding him, not because I couldn't make a decision (well, kind of), but because I found it soothing to look at the colours. If I'm 'fighting' in my head, then that's the perfect time to take the sagging cushions off our old leather sofa and give them a good pounding to bring them back into shape, whereas if I'm in a freeze response then I know I need to come out of it gradually, which is when a warm drink, resting, hugging or going for a walk tend to work a treat.

What's important is to experiment and find out what works for you. Here are some suggestions that my clients have contributed and, as you read them, consider what might feel useful to you, depending on whether you were in fight, flight or freeze mode:

- Talking to a friend
- Walking, running or cycling
- A burst of exercise
- Writing your thoughts and feelings down on paper
- Reading
- Punching pillows
- Lying down and resting
- Listening to your favourite songs
- Vigorous cleaning
- Organising a drawer, desk or cupboard
- Stroking a pet
- Hugging a loved one
- Gentle stretching and movement
- Looking at the sky, trees, a stream or the sea
- Watching reruns of your favourite TV series
- Holding and drinking a warm drink
- Using a hot water bottle or weighted blanket
- Gardening
- Drawing
- Plucking your eyebrows
- Watching funny reels.

Depending on the environment and company you're in, some resources will feel more suitable than others and some might need to wait until you get home at the end of the day, but instead of thinking about all the things you can't do in each situation, find what you can do. And if you really can't do it, imagine yourself doing it or think of a time when you did it – use the power of your mind to create regulating resources.

Embracing the Spectrum of Being Human

We have a natural inclination to seek a regulated state – an equilibrium where we feel connected, capable and resilient. After a stress response, we want to find our way home to regulation, but be mindful that you don't set a conscious or subconscious goal of being regulated all the time. This isn't a realistic or even desirable goal. Being human means experiencing the full spectrum of emotions and responses, including fight, flight and freeze.

If you find yourself demonising or avoiding these primal responses, it's worth exploring why. Perhaps there's a discomfort in feeling anger or a belief that it's unacceptable to be unable to take immediate action. But it's crucial to remember that fight, flight and freeze are not inherently negative or undesirable, just as being regulated isn't inherently 'good'. They are innate survival mechanisms deeply ingrained within us and, instead of viewing them as adversaries to overcome, approach them with curiosity, understanding and gratitude. After all, they're literally keeping you alive.

A regulated state is valuable because it leads to connection with oneself, others and the world around us. It's a space where we can tap into our creativity and curiosity, and pursue our goals with resilience and adaptability. But there are times when our nervous system needs to mobilise, and times when it benefits us to pause and withdraw. Each nervous system state serves a purpose by trying to keep us alive.

Attempting to remain in a constant state of regulation would not only be exhausting, but it would also disconnect us from the richness of the human experience and hinder our connections with others. You might frame it as protecting yourself, but that doesn't mean it's protective or supportive. Something that starts out as protective can become hard, brittle and weak, and not protective at all. No nervous system state is inherently good or bad, each has its place and function, so instead of striving for an unattainable goal of eternal regulation, embrace the ebb and flow of your nervous system responses. By releasing the notion of constant regulation and leaning into the full range of our human experience, you'll open yourself up to the depth of connection, growth and resilience that comes from honouring the wisdom of our nervous system and collaborating with it.

Chapter 4

Boundaries

Boundaries are a sure-fire way to reclaim your power and improve your well-being. They are the unsung heroes of our emotional and physical health. Yet despite their importance, setting and maintaining boundaries can be challenging, and just considering giving a boundary brings up all manner of thoughts and feelings.

Do you feel guilty or selfish for prioritising yourself and being clear about what's okay and not okay? Do you have a looming fear that setting boundaries will lead to disagreements, arguments and, ultimately, damage relationships? Perhaps you weren't taught how to establish boundaries in a healthy way or haven't witnessed positive examples of others communicating their boundaries.

To that, you can add our socialisation. We're socialised from a young age to be nurturing and accommodating, to self-sacrifice and to put the needs of others first – family, children, partners, even complete strangers! If you've been taught to avoid confrontation by being agreeable and polite, then the idea of asserting your boundaries may bring up fear of how the other person will react and feel like the emotional equivalent of climbing Everest. You may also worry about how you'll be perceived – aggressive, selfish, too much – so it's no wonder so many of us swallow it up or that boundaries can feel so loaded. However, although these social norms and expectations can make it harder for women to assert their boundaries, they certainly don't make it impossible. They make them necessary.

Neglecting your boundaries can have serious consequences, including resentment, burnout and even physical illness, so it's not surprising that in recent years personal boundaries have become a hot topic. On the one hand, this has been great, because plenty of people have gone on to create boundaries and honour them, and doing so has benefitted them. Together, we have collectively begun to flex our boundary muscles and that's a very good thing.

On the other hand, though, strengthening one muscle group in isolation creates contraction and tightness, as well as weakness in other areas. In focusing on boundaries like this, everything has become related to boundaries and led to some misunderstanding about what they are – or rather, what they are not – so let's clear that up by going back to basics.

What are Boundaries?

A boundary is a real or imagined line that marks the edge or limit of something. Picture a house with a front garden. Most of the time there will be a clear indication of where one property ends and where another begins, or where private property becomes public space. When I leave my house and walk down the front path, I know that the gate and the wall mark the edge of our property. Similarly, the hedge on the right and the tiny wall on the left are the lines that separate our property from that of our neighbours.

Boundaries are the limits we set for ourselves and others to protect our needs, values and overall sense of self. They are where you end and another person begins; they are the place where you say, 'That's enough, that's my limit.' Boundaries can take many forms; they include establishing physical space between ourselves and others, and communicating in relationships. We all have differing needs, desires and preferences, and what each of us is comfortable with is going to vary from individual to individual.

If our neighbours painted the front of their house and ended up painting some of our house I'd definitely have something to say about it, because it would constitute a boundary transgression. I'd let them know that they'd gone over the invisible line on to our patch and that what they'd done wasn't okay. But believe it or not, there are some people who wouldn't care, so even though a physical and legal boundary had been crossed, it might not be an issue for them. And there are others who wouldn't mind this happening, but would have liked to be asked.

If I didn't say anything to the neighbours, then they might not realise that there's an issue. In fact, they could end up thinking that we like the paint colour and take it upon themselves to paint our house too, all the while thinking that they're doing us a massive favour. It sounds laughable and ridiculous, but this is what happens with boundaries all the time – a boundary is crossed but nothing is said, so the person remains clueless that there's a problem and continues to behave in the same way.

My client Ruby's housemate believed in an 'open-door policy' and would often walk into Ruby's room unannounced for a chat. Ruby was uncomfortable, but never mentioned it, not wanting to seem unfriendly. Her housemate, misinterpreting her politeness as agreement, made her visits a regular occurrence, because she was under the impression that Ruby enjoyed them. When I coached Ruby, she was annoyed at her housemate's lack of consideration and respect for her personal space, but when I asked if she'd been explicit about her needs and preferences, she realised that she'd been expecting her housemate to read her mind and, in doing so, was abdicating responsibility for being clear about her boundaries. As Ruby's frustration softened, what emerged was gratitude and understanding that she had a housemate who wanted to hang out with her.

Lines of connection

Boundaries may seem like barriers that disrupt relationships, but a well-tended one creates connection and healthier relationships. They are a way for us to be clear about how we want to be treated, creating an atmosphere of mutual respect and understanding. This minimises misunderstandings and disappointments.

When you let someone know where your edges are, you're being true to yourself – your needs, desires and values. This authenticity is key to genuine connections with others and your willingness to show your authentic self encourages others to do the same. When boundaries are established, respected and upheld, it also builds trust in a relationship; trust that each person can be relied upon to be clear about their limits and to respect the limits of the other person. This respect for each other's individuality and personal space strengthens the bond between individuals, creating a secure connection and opportunities for ongoing communication.

Over time, a lack of boundaries in a relationship, on the other hand, can lead to disconnection. You might find yourself frequently sacrificing your needs for the sake of others, leading to feelings of resentment as you may feel unappreciated or taken for granted. In relationships without boundaries, it's easy to lose sight of your own interests, desires and identity. This loss can produce a sense of disconnection, not only from yourself, but also from the relationship. Add to that taking on too much emotional, physical or mental load, which can lead to exhaustion or burnout, which, in turn, can result in a desire to distance yourself from the relationship.

A lack of boundaries can send a signal to the other person that they can behave in any way they please, even if it's disrespectful. This lack of respect can lead to a sense of disconnection and an imbalance in the relationship, with one party doing more of the work or making more of the sacrifices, so one or both parties end up feeling undervalued or exploited. In relationships without boundaries, there is a risk of one party becoming manipulative or controlling. This dynamic can create a hostile environment, leading to disconnection.

Setting boundaries is a crucial part of maintaining healthy relationships, but as you'll discover in this chapter, they don't have to be the heavy, big conversations that you anticipate them being.

Crossing the Line

Boundaries serve as invisible lines of respect and understanding. They are the guidelines that define how we want to be treated and what we consider acceptable behaviour from others, but these boundaries can sometimes be crossed or violated, leading to discomfort, conflict and even harm. These violations, known as boundary transgressions, can take various forms and can occur in different areas of our lives, including:

- Physical: Standing too close to someone in a way that makes them uncomfortable, unwanted touching, or entering someone's personal space without permission (for instance going into someone's room without knocking).
- Emotional: Dismissing or invalidating someone's feelings, belittling, criticising them excessively, or trying to control or manipulate their emotions.
- Privacy: Reading someone's personal messages or emails without permission, sharing personal information about someone without their consent, or not respecting someone's wish for solitude or alone time.
- Time: Expecting someone to be available at all times, not respecting someone's personal time, or consistently being late for appointments or commitments.
- Intellectual: Dismissing or belittling someone's ideas or opinions, stealing ideas and presenting them as your own in meetings, copying someone's work without giving them credit, or not respecting someone's intellectual property rights.

- Financial: Manipulating someone into lending money, not repaying borrowed money, accessing someone else's accounts or using their phone to pay for things without permission. These actions are also illegal.

Boundary transgressions can be obvious or subtle and they aren't always intentional – many boundary transgressions are the result of someone being well-intentioned – but this is why it's so important to express when you're not okay with something.

Drawing the Line

Nobody else is in charge of your boundaries. Nobody else has the right or ability to govern your boundaries, it is on you to communicate and uphold them. It is understandable to wish that other people were instinctively aware of any boundary transgressions, because it would spare you the potential discomfort of having to articulate what's unacceptable to you. However, when a boundary transgression happens, it is not the responsibility of the other person to magically know that a transgression has taken place, it is yours.

Upholding boundaries can be a daunting task as it involves a level of risk; the risk of confrontation, disagreements, fall outs or even rejection. Rather than risk this happening, you might choose to overlook the transgression, but the issue does not simply dissolve. Instead, it continues to brew, cultivating feelings of resentment, bitterness and creating a disconnection. This is likely to lead to a deeper rift than if the matter had been addressed head-on.

My suggestion is to embrace the unfamiliarity, the awkwardness and the discomfort that comes with honouring your boundaries, because you can either feel them now while taking a course of action that serves you or you can brace yourself for an even more uncomfortable situation down the line, when you haven't expressed your boundaries and months, years, or even decades have elapsed.

Setting boundaries can be uncomfortable, especially when you first start flexing your boundary muscles, but the alternative (a brewing pot of resentment and disconnected relationships) is much more damaging in the long run. The discomfort of setting boundaries is a momentary feeling; the fallout from not doing so can last a lifetime. Choose wisely.

Client Story

My client Georgie found herself in a situation where her own needs and the needs of her family were not being respected by a well-intentioned, but overeager, family member.

In the beginning, they agreed on a specific time frame for visits in order to accommodate the baby's nap schedule. However, when the family member began arriving at other times, Georgie didn't mention that this didn't suit them. She'd let them in with a smile, but inside she was seething. Instead of communicating the boundary clearly, she hid from the situation – sometimes even physically hiding from view to avoid confrontation. As time wore on, her frustration grew and she found herself blaming the family member, recounting the situation to friends and replaying it in her head. All the while, the family member remained oblivious to the problem, happily arriving at the door and being welcomed in (or under the impression that everyone was out).

Georgie's inability to communicate the boundary was rooted in fear; fear of discomfort, fear of upsetting the family member, fear of disconnection. She was under the impression that boundaries would create distance in the relationship, but in reality it was her failure to set those boundaries that led to disconnection. Through coaching, she came to understand that boundaries are not weapons like 'spears and rifles', but protective measures like 'hedges and fences'. They aren't about punishment or shame, but about self-respect and love for others. By failing to set boundaries, she missed an opportunity to deepen her relationship with her family, while also honouring her own needs and preferences. Whether in family relationships or other areas of life, clear and compassionate boundary setting is key to maintaining healthy connections with others.

Access granted

Another way of thinking about boundaries is to consider levels of access and who gets access to what. Most people walking down our street don't come into our garden. A small number will come up the path and to our front door. Of those, some will step inside the hallway and some will be invited further inside to the living areas. An even smaller number will be allowed to hang out upstairs and it's exceedingly rare for anyone to be in our bedroom. Access depends on who, what, where and when, and so do your personal boundaries.

Those closest to you have a different amount of access to you than someone you barely know, and what's accepted and expected probably fluctuates depending on the person and the situation. I'm guessing that you wouldn't be okay if a stranger came up to hug you on the street, whereas if you bumped into a close friend you might be open to hugging them. My son has extensive access to me – physically, emotionally and practically – but there's no way that I'd give him access to my online accounts, especially after a series of unexpected parcels arrived at our house, because he'd figured out how to use my Amazon Prime account. You might be willing to be in the bathroom at the same time as your sister, but baulk at the idea of being in there with your romantic partner (or vice versa).

You can be exceedingly close to someone and still have very firm boundaries – being in a relationship doesn't mean your boundaries have to dissolve. My partner Paul and I have been together for 10 years and we have a huge amount of respect for each other's boundaries. We don't have to remind each other of them, so they are unspoken but ever present.

Too Close for Comfort

Close families and relationships are hugely beneficial and can be a great thing. When close relationships are healthy, they are supportive, but also allow for differences between individuals, and physical and emotional boundaries exist. There is a bond and a family, couple or friendship can function as a unit, but each member also has their own life; they can enjoy time together and time apart, for example. An enmeshed relationship, though, is like a tightly woven tapestry, where the threads of individuality and boundaries become blurred, intertwining and obscuring the true essence of each person involved. It is a state of emotional fusion, where the lines between one's own thoughts, desires, feelings and beliefs become entangled with those of another, resulting in a loss of autonomy and self-identity. Personal boundaries become blurred or erode away entirely, and individual needs and wants end up taking a backseat to the demands and expectations of the other person. The distinction between 'you' and 'me' becomes hazy, and decisions are made together, often at the expense of personal fulfilment.

This type of relational pattern can arise as a result of familial dynamics, early attachment experiences or a fear of abandonment. Enmeshment often stems from a deep longing for connection and love, but, unfortunately, it can lead to emotional suffocation and a stifling of personal growth. Signs of enmeshment include:

- Lack of appropriate boundaries, including privacy: In enmeshed relationships, there is little distinction between personal space, thoughts and emotions. What's felt by one is felt by all and there may be intrusiveness.
- Excessive emotional dependency: One or both individuals in the relationship may rely heavily on the other for emotional support and validation. They may struggle to regulate their own emotions independently and look to their partner for constant reassurance and validation. A parent may be emotionally dependent on their child and refer to them as their best friend, rather than maintaining a parental relationship.
- Difficulty making decisions: Decision-making can be challenging and anxiety-inducing. There may be a constant need to consult with or seek approval from the other person before making even minor choices, and a fear of disappointing or upsetting them, especially if it involves going against the grain of the done thing within a family or relationship. Individuals may struggle to identify what they want or, if they do know, feel unable to voice it out of fear of how it will be received.
- Loss of personal identity: Individual identities become overshadowed by the relationship and one or both partners may struggle to identify their own values, interests and goals independent of the relationship. It can feel like every aspect of your life must be shared with the other person. Parents can be over-involved in their adult children's lives, often requesting information and updates, and interfering in independent activities and relationships. Emotional manipulation and guilt-tripping behaviours can also be used as a way of exerting control.
- Sacrificing personal needs: One or both individuals may feel responsible for a parent, friend or partner's well-being, and prioritise maintaining harmony and meeting the other person's expectations, even if it means neglecting their own well-being.
- Emotional enmeshment: This occurs when the emotions of one person heavily influence the emotions of the other. There may be a strong

emotional fusion, where it becomes difficult to distinguish between each individual's emotions and experiences.

- An inability to tolerate conflict and tension in the relationship: The fear of upsetting or losing the other person can lead to avoiding or suppressing conflict, resulting in unresolved issues, resentment and a lack of healthy boundaries and communication.

Breaking free from enmeshment requires a conscious effort to re-establish boundaries and develop a stronger sense of individual identity. It involves recognising and honouring one's own needs and desires, even if they differ from the expectations or desires of the other person. As many of my clients have found, it's challenging and uncomfortable, but revolutionary. When my client Leanne decided to accept a job offer in a different city to the one she'd grown up in, her parents took it personally and told her that she was running away and that she didn't care about them. While they were right about her trying to get away and live her own life by putting some physical distance between herself and them, they were wrong in their assumption that it meant she didn't care. In fact, she cared deeply about them, but she had decided to care about herself, too.

Caught in the Net

Enmeshment refers to the blurring of boundaries (or a lack of them) and the loss of individual identity within a relationship. Individuals in an enmeshed relationship may have difficulty distinguishing their feelings, needs or thoughts from those of the other person. This intense interconnectedness can lead to a lack of autonomy, independence and an inability to function separately.

While enmeshment might lead to reliance on each other for emotional support and validation, it's not always rooted in a lack of self-esteem or characterised by controlling behaviour. The connection might be born out of shared values, intense affection or other positive aspects, but it can get in the way of personal growth and individual identity.

Co-dependency often arises within enmeshed relationships, as the lack of taking care of personal needs and emphasis on meeting the needs of the other person can create a pattern of enabling and caretaking. In a co-dependent dynamic, one person takes on a caretaker role, constantly seeking to please and rescue the other, even at the expense of their own well-being. This can lead to them deriving their sense of self-worth from being needed. In relationships, one or both parties can be co-dependent.

Co-dependency is characterised by a pattern of behaviour where one person's self-esteem and functioning are linked to taking care of another person, often to the detriment of their own needs. It often emerges in relationships where one person is dealing with an addiction or chronic illness and the other person takes on the caregiver role.

In both enmeshment and co-dependency, both individuals can become reliant on each other for emotional support and validation, struggling to function independently. However, not all enmeshed relationships are co-dependent, and not all co-dependent relationships are necessarily enmeshed. Enmeshment often involves an intense emotional connection and blurred boundaries, without necessarily involving unhealthy caregiving or control dynamics, whereas co-dependency is typically characterised by a pattern of caregiving that can lead to neglect of one's own needs, often connected to addiction, illness or other chronic issues in one of the partners.

Parentification refers to the reversal of the parent-child relationship. Instead of receiving emotional and practical support, the child is expected to provide it to the parent, taking on excessive levels of responsibility and interrupting the maturation process. This phenomenon adds another layer to the complex dynamics of family relationships, further highlighting the importance of clear boundaries and healthy communication.

Handshakes and Spanks

Personal boundaries aren't a set of fixed rules that apply uniformly to every individual and situation. They are dynamic, evolving constructs that vary depending on all sorts of factors, including a person's comfort level, cultural background, environment, relationships and the specific context in which they find themselves. What might be considered a normal interaction in one setting could be viewed as a transgression in another. Recognising and respecting these shifting boundaries requires an understanding of how different environments and circumstances can influence what is deemed acceptable or inappropriate behaviour.

When I meet someone for the first time, I like to shake their hand, but I have friends who usually go in with a hug and others who prefer not to have physical contact of any kind. The amount of personal space around you and the level of physical contact you're willing and wanting to have with someone else varies from person to person, but some boundaries will also change depending on the environment and circumstances – there might be some topics that you're up for talking to colleagues about in the pub on a Friday night, but which you wouldn't feel comfortable discussing in a Monday morning meeting.

If someone were to slap me, that would be unacceptable and constitute a boundary transgression, and I imagine that it would be to you as well. You probably also don't go around slapping others. But if you're a consenting adult who takes part in BDSM (bondage, dominance/discipline, submission and masochism), then there may be times and situations in which you consent to being slapped or spanked, or when you'll slap and spank someone else.

In a professional workplace, there might be expectations for formal attire and showing up in casual wear might be seen as a violation of the unspoken dress code. However, the same outfit might be perfectly appropriate at a casual weekend gathering with friends. The boundary of what is considered acceptable clothing can shift depending on the setting and the social norms of that environment.

While it might be acceptable and even encouraged to share personal life stories and emotions with close friends or family members, doing the same with a new acquaintance or at a professional networking event might be considered overstepping a boundary. The level of intimacy and trust in the relationship, as well as the context of the conversation, can greatly influence what is deemed appropriate to share.

Not all boundaries are static, some are fluid and context dependent. Understanding and respecting these shifting boundaries are essential for effective communication and healthy relationships in various social situations.

Accidental transgressions

Boundary transgressions can happen by accident, because the other person isn't aware of where your edge is. In fact, you may not be sure of your limits yourself until someone does something that helps you to see where they are, usually by going beyond what is acceptable to you. Boundary transgressions can also happen when someone is being well-intentioned. It's crucial to bear these two things in mind, because often when our boundaries are transgressed we can be so busy being mad at the other person that we forget that their actions are well-intentioned or they just have no idea that what they're doing is a problem, usually because we haven't actually told them!

Approaching accidental boundary breaches with compassion and understanding is usually beneficial to all parties – remember that not all transgressions need to be staunchly defended! Most people don't purposefully intend to cause unease or harm, but that doesn't mean we should simply sweep these moments under the rug, because they can be opportunities to articulate your boundaries, to learn and grow from the experience, and improve your communication skills.

Client Story

By taking an opportunity to communicate a boundary you're not just reacting to a specific problem, but proactively establishing healthier boundary dynamics for the future. Take, for instance, my client Katie's experience with her partner and the issue of unexpected guests: 'I communicated a boundary with my partner, who is totally fine with surprise guests, but I am not. I asked that he give me notice if someone is coming over, even if it is only 10 minutes. He has taken this in his stride and made me feel much more confident in speaking up about any boundaries in future, but I realise that even if he didn't do this, I still communicated my boundary successfully.'

When you are congruent in communicating what is and isn't okay for you, you not only model to yourself that it's okay for you to do so, but you also bring that congruency and authenticity into your personal and professional relationships.

Client Story

As she explains, my client Ulrike found she needed to communicate a boundary in her place of employment: 'I usually fill in for my head of department at certain meetings whenever she isn't available to attend herself. On one occasion she told the person organising a meeting that I would be replacing her on a certain day without asking me if I would be available. I wasn't happy about that and after some preparation about how and what exactly I wanted to say, I set a boundary and told her I would be happy to fill in for her, but only if I don't have any other meetings or responsibilities at that time, and therefore she should check in with me first before deciding over my time and making commitments on my behalf.

'Looking back, it went really well, but the conversation was really tricky for me. My head of department wasn't happy. She got quite defensive and told me that I was overreacting. I told her that I accepted her opinion, but that we would need to agree to disagree. I emphasised that she should please check in with me first and she hesitantly agreed. Two months later, she couldn't attend a meeting and sent me a quick message asking if I could cover for her. I happily agreed to do it.'

In these stories, the underlying lesson is the same: recognising, communicating and respecting boundaries is an evolving journey that, when approached with clarity and empathy, benefits both parties.

Red Flags

Recognising when someone has crossed a personal boundary can be obvious and intuitive for some, but it may take more introspection for others. Likewise, some boundary transgressions will be obvious and instantly identifiable to you, and others could feel murky, requiring reflection and perhaps discussion with loved ones or trusted professionals. Signs that may indicate your boundary has been crossed include:

- Emotional reactions: You might feel discomfort, anger, resentment or anxiety. These feelings are often your body's way of signalling that something isn't quite right.

- Physically pulling away: If you don't actually recoil, you may feel the urge to do so or you may experience other bodily changes, such as an uneasy feeling in your stomach or a tightness in your chest. Your body may be reacting in these ways as an instinctual response to the boundary violation.
- Recurrent thoughts: If you can't stop thinking about an interaction or situation, it might indicate that a boundary was transgressed. You may replay the situation in your head, trying to understand what went wrong.
- Feeling disrespected or violated: If you feel disrespected, not listened to, or if the interaction left you feeling violated, these can be clear signs of a boundary transgression.
- Invasion of privacy: If someone is prying into your personal matters, reading your personal messages or entering your private spaces without your express permission, these are all boundary violations.
- Overstepping commitments: If someone is pressuring you into commitments, such as time, money or emotional support, beyond your comfort level or capacity, this could be a boundary issue.
- Discomfort with physical touch: If someone is touching you in a way that makes you uncomfortable or if they're ignoring your cues to stop, they've crossed a physical boundary.
- Feeling drained: If spending time with someone consistently leaves you feeling drained or exhausted, it could be a sign that they're overstepping your boundaries, either by requiring too much emotional labour or by not respecting your need for time and space.
- Guilt and manipulation: If someone is consistently making you feel guilty for not meeting their needs or wants, or if they're manipulating you to do things you're uncomfortable with, they're likely crossing your boundaries.

Some behaviours that violate personal boundaries can escalate into or already constitute abuse. Abuse, whether it's emotional, physical, sexual or psychological, goes beyond the realm of a simple boundary transgression. It's a serious issue that often involves a pattern of behaviour aimed at controlling, manipulating, or causing harm to another person. If you find yourself or someone you know in a situation where boundary violations have escalated to abuse, it's important to seek professional help and support. Protecting your safety and well-being is paramount, and situations of abuse warrant intervention beyond the scope of what's discussed in this book.

Remember, everyone's boundaries are unique and can change based on the relationship or situation. You have the right to establish and enforce your boundaries, and you also have the right to change them as you see fit. However, it is your responsibility to communicate these boundaries clearly to others and take action when they are crossed.

What's Your Response?

Your SRS plays a vital role in how you perceive, establish and respond to boundaries. It's tied closely to our feelings of safety and comfort, and activates our responses when a boundary is transgressed and a red flag is waved. There are a few ways this relationship plays out.

When our boundaries are crossed, our nervous system may activate the fight, flight or freeze response, depending on our past experiences and coping mechanisms. For instance, if someone invades our personal space, we might move away (flight), ask them what their problem is (fight) or become still and not know how to respond (freeze).

Your body may give you somatic responses – physical cues – when a boundary is being infringed upon, even if you aren't consciously aware of it. You might feel a knot in your stomach, increased heart rate, tightness in the chest, or other physical signs of discomfort or anxiety.

For people who've experienced trauma, certain boundary violations might trigger trauma responses. This can lead to heightened stress, anxiety and physical symptoms. For example, if someone with a trauma history is touched without consent, it could trigger a more intense response than in someone without such a history.

The nervous system regulates our sense of safety. When our boundaries are respected, we often feel safe and comfortable, but when they are violated, we might feel threatened or uncomfortable, and our nervous system responds accordingly.

Leaky, Strong or Rigid

If you're monitoring your responses to boundary transgressions, it can be helpful to get in the habit of assessing when your boundaries are leaky, strong or rigid, so imagine a section of your garden fence has blown down or a few small plants haven't yet grown into a sturdy hedge. This is what leaky boundaries look like. They're porous and easily breached. If you have leaky boundaries, you might feel unsure of what you want, struggle to ask for what you need and feel taken advantage of. You might also feel overly responsible for others' feelings. For example, if a friend sends you an excessive number of text messages and voice messages that go beyond what you're up for and you do nothing about it, that's a sign of a leaky boundary.

Strong boundaries are like a well-maintained fence or a fully grown hedge. They're clear to you and, when appropriate, to others as well. They allow you to be yourself and accept others when they are being themselves. These boundaries may also have a degree of flexibility, as there are times when you might choose to temporarily or permanently bend your boundaries. For instance, if a friend asks to meet up after work, but you've had a long day and were looking forward to unwinding, you might choose to set a boundary in terms of your time and your need to unwind. This wouldn't be a boundary transgression; it's just a request that you get to respond to in a way that respects your boundaries.

Rigid boundaries are like a high, impenetrable wall. They require a lot of energy to maintain and can feel tight and restrictive. If you have rigid boundaries, you might find yourself constantly on guard, trying to control others' behaviour towards you, even when it's unnecessary. This can be exhausting and can create a barrier to genuine connection with others.

What isn't a boundary violation

Understanding the nature of your boundaries can help you navigate relationships more effectively and ensure your own well-being, but, while I'm all for the recognition and respect of personal boundaries, understanding what does not constitute a boundary transgression is equally important.

Disagreements, constructive criticism, questions, invitations and requests, and people wanting to talk about topics and clarify things with you are all part of being human. Others have as much right as you do to express their views and opinions, and just because someone doesn't behave in the way that you want them to, it doesn't necessarily mean that they've crossed a boundary. Remember, the goal of setting boundaries is not to control others, but to create a healthy and respectful environment for yourself and those around you.

When You Just Need to Say No

In fact, you probably don't need to state your boundaries as much as you think you need to, because sometimes instead of setting a boundary, you just need to say no. When your boss or a client asks you to do some last-minute work, that's not a boundary transgression, they've just made a request of you and you get to answer as you see fit. If, however, they make this request by behaving inappropriately – yelling at you or physically intimidating you – then that would constitute a boundary transgression and it would call for a response such as, 'If you continue to shout at me like this then I'm going to speak to HR, because I'm not comfortable with what's going on right now.'

Perhaps your boss calls you outside your agreed work hours. If this is something that you're not on board with, then you might choose to communicate a boundary with them and explain what will happen if they continue to do so. For example, you might say, 'I realise that this felt like the best way to contact me, but I'm not available to answer calls outside work hours, so in future I won't answer. If we need to look at improving communication between us and creating time in our schedules to discuss projects, I'm very open to that.'

Most of the time when I hear people talking about work and boundaries, this isn't what they mean. They're usually talking about being clear about the hours they are available to work, starting and leaving work on time and saying no to some requests and projects so that they aren't over-committed and completely overstretched. While each of these do involve you being more boundaried with your time, they don't constitute a boundary transgression. However, they could well be related to people-pleasing and feeling unable to say no (fear not, there's an entire chapter about people-pleasing just around the corner).

Silent Signals

Responses to boundary transgressions will vary depending on the boundary transgression itself as well as the context and environment in which it took place. Although boundaries are a way for you to communicate what you're cool with and what you're not cool with, responding to boundary transgressions doesn't always require words. Non-verbal cues can be powerful communicators too. Moving away or closing off your personal space can signal you are uncomfortable, so you might step back if someone is too close, move to a different location or use shut doors and headphones to signal that you're not available. Body language and facial expressions can also convey disapproval or discomfort – for example, folding your arms and holding a neutral or critical facial expression.

If someone is trying to provoke you or bait you into a response, choosing not to react can send a strong message, too, and in some situations silence can be a potent response. By not engaging in an argument or responding to offensive comments and behaviour, you signal that you won't tolerate it. And, again, sometimes the most effective non-verbal response is to physically leave the situation. This is a clear indicator that a boundary has been crossed and you will not engage further.

These non-verbal cues can be very clear, but often they're most effective when paired with clear verbal communication about your limits, too. If someone consistently crosses yours despite your non-verbal cues, it might be necessary to articulate your boundaries directly and assertively.

I never want to be around anyone who's smoking (yes, I'm a vehement ex-smoker), but if I'm in a public space where smoking is permitted I don't go up to people and berate them for their lifestyle choices, I simply walk away. However, if someone lit up in my house, my response would be completely different, because there's no way that I'm going to leave my own house. I'd let them know that smoking in our home isn't okay and that they should put it out or leave. Whether you need to say something is going to depend on the situation.

I'm in a monogamous relationship and neither of us think it's acceptable for us to flirt with other people. That's a boundary in our relationship, so if I'm out and someone I don't know starts flirting with me, I simply end the conversation and walk away or let them know that I'm not interested. I don't need to come down hard and heavy and let this stranger know about my boundaries. If, however, this person is someone that I know, that requires a different approach; one where I explicitly tell them to stop.

I'm also incredibly sensitive to scent and most perfumes give me a headache, so if I'm on the tube and someone wearing a strong scent gets into my carriage, I usually just change the carriage that I'm in. I don't go up to that person and ask them to get off. If, on the other hand, I am hosting an event and people have invested their time and/or money to attend, then I let everyone know in advance not to wear perfume, and I explain why and how it prevents me from doing my job. I also inform them in advance that if someone does arrive wearing perfume then they'll be asked to leave. By being upfront and explicit, and stating the consequence, I'm able to honour my needs, while also giving people an opportunity to recognise and honour what's best for them.

How to Talk about Boundaries

Ideally, talking about what you're okay and not okay with is part of your usual communication with others, but what about when someone crosses a boundary? Here are some pointers for how to approach the conversation:

- Identify the transgression: The first step in communicating a boundary is to clearly identify what the boundary transgression was. This requires self-awareness and understanding of your own comfort zones and limits.
- Be clear about the consequences: What will happen if the boundary continues to be transgressed? 'If you continue to drive like this then I won't get in a car with you.' 'If you behave this way in future, then I will report you to HR.' 'If you're going to be late, please let me know because if you're more than 15 minutes late and I haven't heard from you, I'm not going to hang around waiting.' This is not about punishing the other person, but about taking responsibility for your own actions and reactions. This step also provides a moment to check in and see if a boundary has actually been crossed or if you just don't like what someone has said or done.
- Use 'I' statements: This puts the focus on your feelings rather than placing blame on the other person. 'I would love it if we took turns speaking.' 'I'm not comfortable with that arrangement, let's try to find another solution.' 'I don't like it when people come over without prior arrangement, even people that I really love and want to see. My preference is that it's something we agree to in advance.'

- Communicate assertively: When stating a boundary, be assertive and direct. You don't need to apologise or explain excessively. Simply state what the boundary is and what the consequence will be if it's not respected.
- Follow through: Most boundaries require follow-through. If the boundary continues to be transgressed, you need to take the action you stated you would.
- Practise emotional resilience: Giving boundaries can be uncomfortable, especially at first. It's important to be willing to experience these emotions and to understand that it's a part of the process of asserting your boundaries.
- Avoid defensiveness: While it's natural to feel defensive when your lines have been crossed, it's important to avoid becoming overly defensive. This can lead to rigidity and a lack of connection with others. If it's a situation where you need to defend yourself, go for it.
- Understand boundaries are not ultimatums: Boundaries aren't about controlling others' behaviour, but about expressing your needs and expectations. They're guidelines for how you want to be treated.
- Be flexible: While it's important to maintain your boundaries, it's also important to be flexible. Boundaries can change based on different situations and relationships, and it's important to be open to adjusting them as needed.
- Express understanding: While you're not apologising for setting a boundary, it's important to show understanding. Recognise that the other person might not have any idea that they have transgressed.
- Invite conversation: Boundaries can create connection, so after expressing your perspective, invite the other person to share theirs.
- Offer respect: Be willing to appreciate their boundaries, needs and preferences. After all, it's a two-way street.

Remember, it's okay to feel awkward during these conversations, but as my client Ulrike found, it's worth it. She told me, 'At first it is really uncomfortable and I used to try to avoid it at ANY cost, but once you practise a little and get the hang of it, it becomes so much easier. I start to see the benefits of it more and more. Yes, it's still uncomfortable and I still do worry about the person reacting in a negative way prior to the conversation, but the benefits you get from boundary setting are just huge.' It might take practice to express your boundaries assertively and without apology, but it's an important skill for maintaining healthy relationships and protecting your well-being.

The Golden Rule

How good are you at appreciating and respecting other people's boundaries? You can't go through the world demanding everyone respect yours without appreciating and understanding other people's boundaries. Here are some ways you can do that:

- Listen carefully: If someone communicates a boundary to you, absorb what they're saying. They are sharing something important about their needs and comfort levels, so validate their feelings and express your understanding.
- Ask questions: If you're unsure about someone's edges, it's okay to ask. This shows that you care about their comfort and are committed to respecting their limits.
- Respect their 'no': They're not obligated to explain or justify it.
- Watch for body language: Not all limits are expressed verbally. Pay attention to non-verbal cues like body language and facial expressions, which can indicate when someone is uncomfortable.
- Apologise for mistakes: If you inadvertently cross someone's boundary, apologise sincerely. This shows that you respect their boundaries and are committed to not crossing them in the future.
- Maintain confidentiality: If someone shares personal information with you, respect their privacy and don't share it with others without their consent.
- Don't pressure or manipulate: It's important not to pressure or manipulate someone into crossing their own boundaries. This kind of behaviour is not only disrespectful, but also harmful.

Boundary Clashes

Boundaries aren't always the neat fences and hedges that we want them to be. Other people's boundaries may not coincide perfectly with the ones that we have and a clash of boundaries can occur when two individuals' boundaries conflict with each other.

Client Story

Ella cherished her quiet time at the weekends. It was her sanctuary – a time to read, listen to music and recharge. The tranquillity of her living space was important to her and she'd found a roommate who was naturally reserved and quiet, so their cohabitation had been harmonious. They shared an unspoken understanding of respecting each other's personal boundaries.

But their calm dynamic began to shift when her roommate's new boyfriend started spending more time at the apartment. Suddenly, the shared living spaces were filled with lively conversations, laughter, and the sounds of television shows and movies. The weekend afternoons that were once Ella's peaceful retreat now echoed with the energetic buzz of the couple. The nights, too, weren't spared. The couple would stay up late, their conversations seeping through the thin walls, disturbing not only Ella's treasured quiet time but her sleep as well.

Feeling her boundary infringed upon, Ella decided to communicate her feelings to her roommate. She expressed how she valued the previous peaceful ambiance of their home and how the change was affecting her. In turn, her roommate shared how it was her space too and she wanted to be able to enjoy her time with her boyfriend. The conversation was an opportunity for both parties to understand and respect each other's boundaries. They agreed on a middle ground: the living room would be a quiet space during weekend afternoons and the couple would shift to the roommate's bedroom in the evenings to ensure Ella got her uninterrupted rest.

Navigating these situations requires communication, compromise and respect for each other's needs. The first step is to acknowledge the conflict, because ignoring it won't make it go away and could lead to bigger issues down the line. Being willing to create a space where it can be discussed, even if you're unsure how to approach or solve it, communicates willingness and respect, as does being patient. If you're unable to compromise or find a solution, consider seeking professional support from a mediator, who can provide guidance and tools for effective communication and compromise.

A Dance of Mutual Trust

We each feel comfortable with different things, but it's vital to be able to verbalise that and to accept that from the other person as well, even though it's not the same way we see it. Awareness of and respect for boundaries creates healthy relationships where we can honour the other person's boundaries and, in turn, have our boundaries respected as well.

One of the most vital steps in relationships is the mutual recognition and respect of boundaries. Each person's life experiences and perceptions are unique, and so are the boundaries they set. What seems trivial or permissible to one individual might be deeply significant to another.

Client Story

Recognising these differences is an essential part of nurturing healthy relationships, as Katie found in her relationship: 'My partner requested that when he's telling me something that I listen and not offer suggestions unless he specifies that he wants them. He said he just wants to be listened to and heard when he's going through something tough. My general reaction is to try and help out, but I've been really trying to just hear him instead of taking away his power, and not trusting that he can and will come up with solutions himself. My brain is trying to make it mean that he doesn't value my opinion, but I know that isn't the case.'

Katie's experience sheds light on the subtle nuances of boundaries. It isn't always about dramatic disagreements or overt invasions of personal space. Sometimes it's about these quieter moments of understanding and restraint – recognising when to speak and when to remain silent, when to step in and when to stand back. Through these small but significant actions we build relationships based on mutual respect and trust, and in doing so we honour the boundaries of those we care about and the bonds between us.

Navigating Familial Expectations

Jessica's relationship with her partner highlighted that there can be a delicate balance between family expectations and individual desires. Her partner was from a close-knit family and was used to frequent family gatherings. Now that they lived closer to them, there was an unsaid expectation that they would go to all of them. Jessica told me that every weekend was a family event and that she was feeling overwhelmed and resentful. Within her own family, she was accustomed to far less frequent gatherings and she much preferred to spend time on her own.

In our coaching session, she was able to look at things more factually. She acknowledged that it wasn't *every* weekend and that she didn't even know if her partner or her family wanted her to be at all the family gatherings. However, in Jessica's mind there was a boundary clash going on and it was taking up a lot of mental real estate – no wonder she was feeling so resentful.

Jessica realised that much of her stress stemmed from her assumptions and internalised expectations rather than any explicit demands made by her partner or her family. Through some honest conversations, they were able to better understand each other's perspectives. Her partner was surprised to hear her feelings, sharing that she never expected her to attend every family gathering and was unaware that this was even causing her stress. They decided to find a balance – Jessica would come to some of the gatherings, particularly important family events, but she'd also skip some.

What might seem like a significant boundary clash can often be addressed through understanding and compromise. Sometimes the boundaries we think are being imposed on us are merely boundaries we impose on ourselves through our perceptions and assumptions. It's always worthwhile actually talking to the other people involved and finding out what their preferences, needs and limits are.

One final thing I want to mention is that when you get used to boundaries, you don't need them as much. This is not because you're a pushover or you've achieved some Zen-like state, but because when you're really clear on everything at your end, and you're honest with yourself and with other people about what you're willing and able to do, you don't find yourself in conflict situations quite so often. You also tend to lose the habit of people-pleasing and running yourself into the ground, which, as we'll see, can only be positive.

Chapter 5

People-pleasing

In a world that often demands us to be everything to everyone, it's easy to lose ourselves in the process. We become masters of the art of people-pleasing, bending over backwards to meet the needs of others, often at the expense of our own. Rewriting this narrative means learning to say no, setting boundaries and prioritising our own needs, while navigating guilt or fear of rejection. This chapter is dedicated to exploring just that.

People-pleasing is a complex behaviour, deeply rooted in our emotional need to be liked and approved by others. It's a survival mechanism that often manifests as a constant 'yes' to requests, an overfilled schedule, and a tendency to put our own needs and desires on the back burner. We may find ourselves apologising excessively, allowing others to make decisions for us and going along with things, even when we disagree with them.

For many of my clients, people-pleasing is more than just the habit of saying yes. It can stem from a state of hypervigilance – a constant alertness to the moods and behaviours of others. It's an attempt to manage what others think and feel about you, and to prevent the emotional or physical escalation that you believe will happen if you don't keep things under control. It involves a fear of getting things wrong or a belief – conscious or subconscious – that parts of us aren't acceptable or welcome. Here are some examples of people-pleasing behaviours:

- Difficulty saying no: Agreeing to requests even when you don't have the time or desire to fulfil them, accommodating others and overextending yourself.
- A crowded schedule: This is the inevitable product of saying yes way more times than you say no.
- Taking responsible for others' feelings: You believe you must keep everyone around you happy and you blame yourself when others are upset.

- Feeling guilty: This could be for a range of reasons, but may well include guilt for not doing enough and guilt for attempting to prioritise your own needs and desires.
- Fearing rejection: A desire to be accepted and liked – and being afraid of what it means or how it will feel if you're not – is also a common trait.
- Apologising often: Even when it's not your fault or responsibility, you find yourself apologising, including when there's nothing to actually apologise for!
- Avoiding conflict: You'll probably go to great lengths to avoid disagreements or confrontations.
- Holding back from expressing personal opinions: Hiding your own preferences or beliefs to align with those of others and going along with other people's ideas and plans.
- Editing and censoring yourself: Just being yourself isn't something you do often, if at all.
- Thinking about what other people think about you: You probably spend a lot of time doing this.
- Feeling uncomfortable if someone is angry with you: You might feel a strong need to mend the situation immediately if you perceive someone is upset with you.
- Doing more than your share of work: Whether at home, work or in friendships, you often take on extra tasks to help others.
- Trying to read other people's minds: This is in an attempt to manage other people's thoughts, feelings and behaviours, and often to try and feel safe.

The Hypervigilant Highway

People-pleasing is a complex phenomenon that's often rooted in early life experiences and family dynamics. It's a learned behaviour that can serve as a coping mechanism in response to neglect, conflict or unpredictability in one's environment. Children who grow up in such environments may resort to pleasing others to gain attention, approval or love, or to avoid conflict and maintain a sense of control in unpredictable situations.

People-pleasing is deeply intertwined with the tendency to read or anticipate the behaviour of others. This sensitivity, often honed to a fine point in people-pleasers, can be a great skill, because it allows for a heightened sense of awareness, empathy and understanding, enabling individuals to connect deeply with others. These skills are hugely advantageous in many situations and professions. However, people-pleasing can lead to a state of hypervigilance, where one is constantly on alert, scanning the environment for cues on how to act or respond (but again, there are some occupations where the ability to do so is invaluable).

This hypervigilance is born out of a need for self-preservation. In many cases, people-pleasers have learned from a young age that their safety, both physical and emotional, is contingent on the moods and whims of those around them, leading to a heightened state of alertness where they're always ready to adapt and shift to keep the peace and maintain harmony. And yes, in case you were wondering, this, too, is highly prized in professional roles that require great awareness, tact and diplomacy. (Although this chapter will largely focus on the detrimental effects of people-pleasing, it's not all bad and it's important to highlight that you can frame these things as skills and use them to your advantage.)

Those who are prone to people-pleasing often identify as empaths – individuals who are highly attuned to the emotions and energy of those around them. They feel deeply and often take on the emotions of others as their own. This heightened sensitivity can make them excellent at anticipating the needs and wants of others, often before the person themself is even aware, but it can also lead to a tendency to prioritise the emotions of others over their own. This is a hallmark of people-pleasing. While empathy is a beautiful and powerful trait, it needs to be balanced with self-care and boundaries. Being able to anticipate the needs of others doesn't mean you always have to meet them. Your feelings, needs and desires are just as important and deserving of attention and care. It's not only okay, but necessary, to prioritise yourself.

Many of my clients come to me feeling exhausted and with the sense that they've taken a backseat to their own life. They know they want to stop people-pleasing and to bring in some boundaries, but lack positive examples of what this looks like in practice.

Modelling is a psychological term that refers to the vicarious learning that occurs through observation and imitation of others. Throughout your life, you've had all sorts of beliefs, attitudes and behaviours modelled to you, like whether you should walk away from or persevere with a relationship or job that's no longer a good fit for you; whether different body shapes, sizes and weights are completely normal or the most awful thing ever; or whether it's acceptable to ask for help or not. And, of course, this translates into negating your own needs and preferences, and people-pleasing, so not sending your food back to the kitchen even though it isn't what you ordered, saying yes to all requests made of you and being there for others at all costs.

Client Story

A powerful example of the impact of modelling – and how it can be counteracted – was shared by Godelieve: 'It was modelled to me that you should always be there for others, even at your own cost. Mainly my mom was always so generous with her time and emotional bandwidth with people at work (she's a pastor) that there was often little left for us at home. In the end she burnt out and never fully recovered. I'm a teacher and it took A LOT to recognise when this showed up for me and I am working hard to do it differently, even telling my students explicitly when I had to dial things down that I needed to make choices if I still wanted a life outside of school – I wanted to model taking care of myself for them and to do it in a loving way.'

Of course, you may not know what you want and need, because you're so accustomed to thinking about what everyone else wants and expects of you, and it's understandable to think that you need lots of strategies and that you need to do a lot to create change. However, that doesn't have to be true at all, because that kind of thinking is a product of *toxic productivity*. The capitalist paradigm pushes the notion that more is better, driving us to chase countless tactics, tools and techniques to improve. However, self-awareness and introspection are much more transformative than this relentless pursuit. Embracing self-awareness challenges the toxic productivity narrative that tells us that we need to do more, achieve more and be more. It invites us to just be – to understand ourselves deeply, recognise our patterns and act from a place of self-acceptance. You don't need an exhaustive list of strategies. Self-awareness is far more potent, as Anne's story illustrates.

Client Story

Anne had been feeling unhappy and stuck, and wanted to make some changes, but lacked examples of what those changes could look like: 'The combination of feeling like others know better, people-pleasing, not knowing my body and my hormones, and spending a lot of time in fight, flight and freeze, kept me in a very toxic relationship, caused me to burn out at work and left me feeling like I had no control over my time, calendar and life. I didn't comprehend how feeling unsafe and unsure of myself caused me to exhaust myself pleasing others. I wasn't listening to my needs. In fact, I didn't have a clue what my needs were. And I didn't have an image or example of what doing that would look like in a healthy way.'

Anne started spotting her automatic thought patterns and instead of letting them run the show, she saw them for what they are – just thoughts. Through tracking her menstrual cycle, she was able to stop feeling scared of it and built a welcoming relationship with her body. Learning about stress responses meant that she could spot them and use them as an opportunity to check in with herself.

I love Anne's story, because it's an amazing example of the power of knowing and understanding yourself, and, as she says, 'I've made so many steps in building a different relationship with myself. Instead of being my own biggest bully, I see things that go wrong as a learning curve, not proof that everything will just always go wrong and be shitty, and that I can't "do life" the way others do or I'm supposed to do it. I ended my shitty relationship!'

The Fourth F

We've already covered the stress responses of fight, flight and freeze, but there's a fourth: fawning. Fawning (also known as please-and-appease), was coined by psychotherapist Pete Walker, a specialist in the field of complex post-traumatic stress disorder (C-PTSD). Fawning develops as a survival mechanism in response to environments that are or feel threatening, stressful or traumatic; situations where the individual feels the need to maintain peace or avoid conflict to ensure their safety or acceptance.

It's a response that's particularly prevalent in individuals who've experienced situations where their well-being was dependent on the moods and behaviours of others. Fawning is what we do when, in the presence of a potential threat, we attempt to get on the good side of the source of the threat to avoid or diffuse conflict.

By anticipating and meeting the needs of others, the individual can avoid conflict, criticism or other negative outcomes. Go to any bar and you're unfortunately likely to see please-and-appease in action. You may have experienced it yourself in this setting, when you or a friend have received unwanted attention from a man and found yourself nodding your head and kind of going along with the conversation, enough to keep them happy while also trying not to put out any encouraging signals and simultaneously sending your friend and the bar staff 'rescue me' looks. Sometimes it feels safest to just smile and hope that they'll go away and leave you alone, but that's what fawning is. And it's so important to understand that, because when you understand that it's a nervous system response, you also drop any judgement or shame that you have for doing it in the first place.

Fawning is related to people-pleasing. Both involve a pattern of behaviour where an individual prioritises the needs, desires or opinions of others over their own. This is often done out of a fear of rejection, conflict or negative consequences. However, while people-pleasing can be a trait that develops in various contexts and can sometimes have positive social implications (like fostering cooperation and harmony), fawning is specifically a survival mechanism that develops in response to trauma. It's a way of managing and navigating relationships that are perceived as threatening or unsafe.

Ask for Angela

In the UK, if you are feeling unsafe, vulnerable or threatened, you can discreetly ask for help in bars, clubs and other venues by approaching staff and asking them for 'Angela'. This code word alerts staff that you need their help with a situation and a trained member of staff will then provide appropriate assistance, such as reuniting you with a friend, getting you a taxi or alerting venue security and/or the police.

Please-and-appease is like a long-term coping mechanism that's used when you have to exist in certain relationships and environments, such as the house you grew up in or the work situation you find yourself in. People-pleasers often start out as parent-pleasers, wanting to keep Mum and Dad happy, because if they are okay, then you can be okay. Please-and-appease is an attempt (often highly successful) to keep ourselves safe by managing other people. It's a response that allows you to navigate situations where there are threats to your physical and/or emotional safety on an ongoing basis, but please-and-appease isn't simply about trauma. It can also develop in homes and environments that we would consider and accept as loving and safe, and it can emerge when we recognise that pleasing others is a way to receive attention, love and praise, which we all have a basic human need for.

There are situations where control and manipulation take place, but the foundation of people-pleasing can also be completely unintentional. If you were the eldest sibling, you might have been told how helpful you are and experienced the reward of helping your mum – who wouldn't want more of the loving approval of a mother? – so rather than always being this awful result of a traumatic upbringing (which it can be), I invite you to see how it can emerge in safe and loving situations as well.

My parents loved me and did their very best, but there were times (just as there are for all of us) when they weren't able to regulate their nervous systems and when I suspect that they didn't know how to be emotional in a way that was safe for them or for me. Little Maisie found that scary and so I got very good at taking care of other people in order to feel safe. This strategy makes sense and it was also highly effective. It's even served me well throughout my career – imagine having a birth doula supporting you in labour who seems to have the ability to read your mind and a coach who picks up on the smallest gestures and details. But the conversation around people-pleasing and fawning rarely highlights the normalcy of it as a response, nor the benefits of it.

People-pleasing Pluses

People-pleasing, while often viewed in a negative light due to its potential for self-neglect and exploitation, can be useful, particularly in the short term. When I asked my clients how people-pleasing has served them, here's what they shared:

- It's kept me safe
- I climbed up the career ladder and made friends
- I got some jobs I wanted
- It meant I could get along with people
- It's helped me to fit in
- I gained lots of contacts
- I have been able to diffuse difficult situations
- I could decrease conflict easily
- I can read other people very well
- I'm alert in social situations.

But while these benefits may offer temporary relief or satisfaction, chronic people-pleasing can lead to long-term issues such as burnout, resentment, loss of identity and unhealthy relationships. It's crucial to balance the desire to please others with self-care and personal boundaries.

Masking

Neurodivergent individuals, such as those with autism or ADHD, often engage in masking, or camouflaging, to fit into neurotypical norms. This can involve suppressing natural behaviours or adopting ones that are deemed more socially acceptable. The motivation behind masking is similar to people-pleasing: a desire for acceptance, to avoid conflict or negative reactions, and a need to blend in with societal expectations in order to be safer.

Masking has a toll, though. It's a form of self-protection, a way to navigate a world that may not fully understand or accept neurodivergent behaviours, but although it can make social interactions smoother, it can also have a negative impact on physical and mental health, causing autistic meltdowns and shutdowns.

In the context of neurodivergence, people-pleasing and masking can often be intertwined. A neurodivergent individual might engage in people-pleasing behaviours as part of their masking, going above and beyond to meet others' needs or expectations in an effort to fit in. This can be particularly challenging, as it adds another layer to the already complex process of navigating social interactions.

It's crucial for neurodivergent individuals to have safe spaces where we can be ourselves without the need for masking or people-pleasing. It's also important for society at large to become more aware, accepting and understanding of neurodivergence – 15–20 per cent of us are neurodivergent – reducing the need for these behaviours. Everyone deserves to be accepted for who they are, without the need to constantly adapt or hide parts of themselves.

Shaped by Social Norms

Female socialisation plays a significant role in shaping people-pleasing tendencies. From a very young age, we are taught, both overtly and subtly, a set of social norms and expectations that emphasise agreeableness, nurturance and compliance. Traits like agreeableness, passivity and cooperation are valued in girls. Over time, this can lead us to prioritise others' feelings and needs over our own and make us feel it's important to maintain 'harmony' (at least on the outside), even at the expense of our own well-being.

Women are usually seen as the primary caregivers. As girls, we receive toys like dolls and playsets that mimic household chores, reinforcing the notion of caregiving roles and leading to an internalised belief that our primary value is in caring for others, sometimes to the detriment of caring for ourselves. We're encouraged to be nice, polite and not to make a scene or a fuss. This can create a reluctance to assert preferences and boundaries as adults for fear of conflict or of being perceived anything from fussy to aggressive.

As part of unwinding this socialisation, my client Hannah has been paying attention to the ways in which this can arise. This is what she came up with:

- *'When the hairdresser asks if the water temperature is okay, and I say yes, even though it isn't, because I don't want to make a fuss.*
- *'When I'm in a social setting with a group of people and someone turns to me and asks what I feel like doing and my mind goes blank and I look to other people in the group for clues as to what they might feel like doing – it can feel easier to try to interpret their needs rather than tune into my own.*
- *'When I'm sitting on a train or plane and I really need to pee, but I'm on the inside seat and there's someone next to me and they're deep in their book, listening to something, and I don't want to bother them, so I hold it in and sit*

really uncomfortably for the rest of the journey, or wait until they get up to pee and just go then.

- 'When I'm in a café and they give me the wrong order and I just eat it anyway, because I don't want them to have to remake it.'

Media, family, peers and other societal forces place a high value on our appearance and likability, resulting in a constant need for external validation and an eagerness to please others to receive positive reinforcement. Instead of being praised for showing initiative and leadership, or admired for our ability to be explicit about what we need and want, we're labelled as bossy, aggressive, controlling or selfish when we stand up for ourselves or assert our needs.

We're also taught to derive our self-worth from relationships, whether familial, platonic or romantic. This leads to a belief that we must always accommodate and please others in order to maintain these relationships and our sense of self. We are continuously portrayed as self-sacrificing figures who put family and community needs above their own, adding another layer of pressure to conform and please. Caring for others is wonderful, but you are worthy regardless of what you do (or don't do) for them. You do not need sacrifice yourself in order to take care of everyone else. It's time we unwound this unhelpful socialisation.

Beware of labelling

Unearthing the behaviour of people-pleasing can be enlightening. As Katie points out, naming it has been transformative: '*I know that in the past I have put others' needs before my own, but not been aware of what it was. Giving it a name has brought my attention to it, so I can see when I am doing it and when I'm not.*' Charlotte, another client, echoes this sentiment: '*I always thought there was something really wrong with me and I was the only one in this, but when I found it has a name that many people refer to, I feel like I am not as crazy as I thought.*'

However, it's crucial to differentiate between recognising a pattern of behaviour and solidifying it as an inherent identity. Be wary of adopting the term 'people-pleaser' as a defining aspect of your being. Doing so risks making the behaviour even more ingrained, as if it's an immovable part of your essence.

How you articulate your feelings and behaviours makes a difference. When you describe yourself as an anxious person, you affirm that you are anxious, whereas if you state that you feel anxious, that acknowledges how you feel, while also leaving space for you to feel differently. Similarly, rather than stating, 'I'm a people-pleaser,' perhaps try, 'I've noticed that I people-please in certain situations.' This slight shift in language can make a world of difference, offering more room for change and growth.

If you catch yourself thinking that curtailing people-pleasing is too challenging, because it's 'just how I am,' you're setting a self-imposed limit. These beliefs can stop you from even trying to change or, worse, trap you in the misconception that there's a deeper, unsolvable issue at play.

Tackling people-pleasing tendencies is an evolving journey. I've personally navigated and reduced my people-pleasing tendencies in all sorts of areas of my life and it still crops up. It's almost like I've been socialised into it for four decades **eyeroll**. This is why acceptance – recognising that there might be instances when we revert to old patterns, but without self-critique – is so important. It's not about reaching a definitive endpoint, just noticing these tendencies, dialling them down and recalibrating.

Doubling down on 'I'm fine'

Sometimes, people-pleasing goes unnoticed by those around you, but others pick up on it, asking questions, such as, 'Are you sure about that?' that give you a second chance to be honest. Interestingly, when faced with these opportunities, people-pleasers find themselves instinctively doubling down on their original response. Rather than taking a moment to pause, reflect and answer honestly, they end up emphasising their unwavering ability to fulfil the request or meet the expectation.

The inclination to double down on the original response stems from the activation of the stress response. In moments of stress our focus narrows and we become fixated on finding a single solution or course of action. This narrow focus limits our ability to explore alternative options or consider the implications of our commitments, so when someone questions a people-pleaser's ability or willingness to meet a request, they often dismiss the doubt without truly considering the consequences.

This automatic response not only perpetuates the people-pleasing cycle, but also inhibits the person from recognising the choices available to them.

By disregarding the inquiry and stubbornly affirming their ability, they may unknowingly overlook the opportunity to evaluate their own desires, needs and limitations. In doing so they inadvertently sacrifice their own well-being and may find themselves having to rearrange their entire lives to fulfil the expectations they've committed to. By recognising the activation of the stress response, you can consciously choose to step back from automatic reactions like these and give yourself a chance to consider alternative responses.

The Power of Pausing

Overcoming people-pleasing starts with recognising the urge to please others and understanding the nervous system's response to perceived threats, even if they're just ones that your mind has created. When the nervous system perceives a threat, whether it's fear of conflict, rejection or the potential for discomfort, it can make it challenging to do the things you want to do. When someone makes a request of you, follow these simple steps:

1. Notice if you feel compelled to say yes to try and get out of any discomfort that you're experiencing at that moment.
2. Name the urge for yourself by internally saying, 'I've got an urge to say yes.'
3. Let them know you need to think about it for a moment.
4. Sit with the urge and get to know it. How does it feel in your body and why is it there? What's really going on?
5. Find out what you really want to answer by asking, 'What would I say if I had no fear of repercussions?'
6. Decide how you want to answer and say it out loud. That doesn't mean your answer to point 5 will be the one that you give. There may be times when you determine that you're going to stick with your original response, but you'll be doing so consciously and intentionally, and that's completely different.

That's it. The beauty of this strategy lies in its simplicity. If you just do these things, your life will be forever changed (but I've got other options for you as well). Taking a moment to pause and reflect allows us to resist the automatic urge to please and consider our own needs and desires. By consciously pausing, we create space to evaluate whether saying yes is what we want to say. And sometimes it will be. Lorna's experience is an example of the strategy in action.

Client Story

'I was collaborating on a project at work and a colleague suggested an approach that I wasn't comfortable with. Immediately, my stomach knotted up with anxiety. I was worried about voicing my reservations as I didn't want to appear confrontational or jeopardise our working relationship. My immediate response was to nod in agreement, but remembering the importance of pausing, I took a deep breath and said, "I need a moment to think about it." Giving myself this moment allowed me to reflect on my true feelings and I realised that my initial agreement was driven by fear of conflict rather than the merit of the idea itself. When we resumed discussing it, I was straightforward in expressing my concerns and, to my surprise, my colleague was receptive. We found a middle ground that worked for both of us.'

Working with Your Body

Being in a stress response makes it more challenging (or even impossible) for us to do the things that we want to do. This is why understanding and tending to your nervous system is so important, because if your nervous system is going, *'Hey, it's not safe. It's not safe for you to have needs here. Don't speak up about them, because we don't know what's going to happen, so it's best if we just keep quiet,'* then it's going to be very hard for you to speak up, even if you want to.

If your nervous system is telling you that it's unsafe to do something, then that will trump everything else, because its job is to keep you alive. Trying to strong-arm yourself into thinking differently without addressing your nervous system is unlikely to work. It also won't feel good (does being forced to do something ever feel good?) and it can reinforce unhealthy patterns of behaviour.

Another effective strategy is to experiment with changing posture in response to requests. Simply standing up when someone makes a request can have a profound impact on our confidence and assertiveness. It helps us embody a more empowered stance and sends a subtle signal to both ourselves and others that we are willing to prioritise our own needs.

When I find myself in please-and-appease, I notice that I arrange my body so that it's smaller; my posture conveys an 'I'm no threat to you' vibe or, in a more confronting situation, it's as if I'm trying to go unnoticed, employing the *freeze* response. In that moment, just assuming a different posture makes a difference. Instead of sitting in a hunched-over position that makes you physically smaller, try sitting more upright or expanding your posture in some way. It doesn't have to be as big a change as standing up – expand your chest, become more upright, and wiggle your toes and fingers to create space and safety for yourself to remind your body and brain that you're alright.

Nice for What?

Being kind and being nice, while often used interchangeably, are not the same thing. The difference lies in the depth and intention behind our actions. When we choose to be nice, we focus on being polite, agreeable and maintaining a pleasing demeanour towards others. It may feel comfortable and rewarding, especially if we have been praised for our ability to make others feel good and prioritise their needs. In the short term, being nice may feel like a relief, because in your mind you think you've avoided a potential conflict, but if we zoom out and look at the longevity of a personal or professional relationship, it will have negative consequences and often results in an actual conflict.

Imagine that a colleague asks you for feedback on a project they've been working on and as you review their work, you find some areas where, in your opinion, their work hasn't quite hit the mark or is way off. Rather than saying, 'You know, that work that you did wasn't to your usual standard,' and then having a helpful conversation about it, you opt for minimising the truth or saying nothing, which is not helpful to you or to them. This is being nice in action and it means that you avoid the discomfort that may come from being honest with someone else. Instead, you might tell them that they're doing a great job, even when they aren't, and hold back on communicating clearly and honestly with them. Being nice might sound good to you (and maybe to the other person too), but although those words might sound nice, they're not genuine.

You could do this out of concern about hurting the other person's feelings or because you find it challenging to take part in any conversation that feels slightly confrontational, so instead you opt for taking care of your emotional well-being by trying to manage their thoughts and feelings. But what starts off as trying to be nice to someone ends up being unkind, because it denies them the opportunity to learn and grow, impedes their ability to succeed in their role and can end up causing harm to your relationship with them as colleagues, not to mention not seeing them as capable human beings.

Being kind goes beyond surface-level politeness. Kindness is rooted in generosity, helpfulness and genuine consideration for others' feelings. It involves acting from a place of benevolence, even if it may not always feel comfortable to you to do so. Being kind means providing feedback that genuinely helps someone succeed in their role and grow in their abilities.

Niceness is about surface-level politeness, often motivated by a desire to be liked and accepted or to avoid conflict. It's about maintaining a pleasant facade to avoid rocking the boat, even if it means suppressing your own feelings or needs. This is where it ties into people-pleasing. For a variety of reasons, people-pleasers often default to being nice, even when it's at the expense of their own well-being.

The idea of confrontation or conflict can be extremely distressing and not something they have healthy experiences of. They may have a deep-seated fear of rejection or abandonment and, by always being nice and accommodating, they hope to avoid the potential for being disliked or left out. Society often values politeness and harmony, and for those socialised as female, there is added pressure to be agreeable and nurturing. Being nice is often seen as a virtue, and deviating from this can lead to potential judgement and criticism. Those who struggle with self-worth may believe that their needs, desires, opinions and feelings are less important than those of others, and being nice serves as a way to gain validation or approval from those around them.

In the context of people-pleasing, the shift from being nice to being kind is a crucial one. It entails switching from fear-based decision-making (fear of rejection, fear of conflict) to a place of love and respect for both yourself and others, and understanding that you can care for others without sacrificing yourself.

Being kind might feel harder, because it requires honesty and that can feel risky, especially if you're used to being nice and trying to please others. But it's helpful. Your colleague may not agree with your feedback and they may not use it, but they hopefully walk away from that interaction knowing that you see them as an equal and are willing to say things that might be uncomfortable for you, for their benefit (though, of course, you have no say over how they might interpret your words and behaviour).

Being kind is honest and it's more valuable. Whether someone pays any mind to what you say or not, it's interactions like these that allow us to experience true connections with ourselves and with others. It's how you learn that you are amazing and worthy exactly as you are. You don't have to pretend to be anything or anyone other than yourself, and when you do this work, it is incredibly freeing.

Tone Policing

The other problem with being nice is in how it relates to tone policing, which is a defensive and diversionary tactic that's used when someone doesn't like the content of what another person is saying. They don't like the words that are being spoken, so what they do is draw attention to the way in which those words were said; the tone in which they were said. Being told to calm down or that there's no reason to get so upset or angry are examples of tone policing. In doing so the individuals policing the tone of the conversation seek to establish their authority while dismantling the credibility of those who are labelled as emotional, irrational and unreasonable.

Tone policing is a subtle act of violence that's frequently and regularly experienced by Black women when they're told to *calm down* and *stop being so angry and aggressive*. They're told that if they spoke in a nicer tone, then what they're saying would be better received. And that's extremely problematic for many reasons: it exacerbates the marginalisation and silencing of Black women's experiences and concerns, stereotypes of being angry or aggressive are weaponised against them and it is used to make justifiable anger or frustration seem like an overreaction or irrationality. By emphasising how Black women should express themselves and behave, tone policing diverts the topic of conversation. It's a way of muting Black women's voices, avoiding addressing systemic issues and maintaining control through oppression.

Each person's journey towards self-awareness, acceptance and personal growth is unique. Overcoming deeply ingrained habits, self-judgements and societal expectations can be a challenge that feels insurmountable. But with the right tools and guidance, it is possible to break through these barriers and to do things in a way that's in line with your values, desires and strengths. Evelien's transformation is a testament to this. When she first joined my membership, Powerful, she was trapped in a cycle of stress, perfectionism and external pressures. But as you'll see from her own words, with introspection and tailored strategies, Evelien managed to redefine her relationship with herself, her work and the world around her.

Client Story

Evelien started working with me because she was experiencing work-related burnout, stress and perfectionism. She felt unhappy and unhealthy, and her inner critic was running the show. She judged herself a lot and lived life from a place of what she should do, and as a result, she felt stuck. Evelien was able to recognise what wasn't working, but didn't have the tools to make changes. I asked her what helped:

'Recognising how I often function in an activated stress response state – just noticing makes a big difference. All of this makes me be much more emphatic with my own behaviour and thoughts. Working on more self-acceptance and self-love, instead of all the "should-ing" and perfectionism, has made a big difference.

'I have changed the way I think about my goals and career, have accepted a different path, and not going with what I "should" do. I have taken a lot of action on this: quit a job and started a new platform myself, which is something that I had been wanting to do for years. This now already feels totally logical.

'I have a lot more self-confidence. Some things I was unsure about a year ago I can't even imagine anymore. I approach work and connect to people around work in a more authentic way. This has already created a lot of opportunities and interesting conversations. Part of my issue was I didn't feel seen. I now let myself be seen in a much more connecting and open way, and am not trying to prove myself all the time anymore.

I have already proven myself. I know my worth. I feel a lot less guilt and do a lot less "should-ing". Now I have a lot more clarity about why I do and feel things, which makes things feel less complicated. I have more joy, ease and spaciousness.

'I embraced what I really like and my need to be alone a lot, without my partner and son. And I also really get energised from meeting people if I can get into meaningful conversations. I am not so good at small talk. I let my partner handle this, as he is a star at it. I don't let this mean anything about me.'

I Have To...

Once you remove 'I have to' and 'I need to' you might discover that you actually want to do many of these things. Just because something you do could be described as people-pleasing, it doesn't mean it's always people-pleasing – it all depends on where it's coming from.

1. Write a list of all the things you do because you think you have to. Attending your niece's birthday party, going out with a friend to their favourite spot, that work project, coffee with your colleague, having your in-laws stay with you... What are all the little and large roles and responsibilities that feature in your life?
2. Keep the list somewhere that's easy for you to access and add to in the moment –the notes app on your phone or a notebook that you carry around with you is perfect.
3. Every time you catch yourself saying I need to, I ought to or I have to, stick it on your list. Seeing how much you do (or don't do) is enlightening and many of my clients have been shocked to see the extent of their lists.
4. After a few weeks of adding to your list, it's time to assess it.
5. Picture me taking your list and either ripping it up or burning it. Are there any items on your list that you'd want to keep? Because while there are things that you tell yourself you *have* to do, you may also *want* to do them. In which case, you just need to change your thoughts about them, so that you don't feel weighed down by obligation and dread.

Unplugging from the Approval Matrix

At the heart of people-pleasing behaviour often lies a deep-seated belief about one's self-worth. Many people-pleasers struggle with low self-esteem and a sense of their own value that is heavily dependent on the approval and validation of others. This can lead to a cycle where the individual constantly seeks out external validation in order to feel good about themselves, often at the expense of their own needs and desires.

This cycle can be self-perpetuating. The more you engage in people-pleasing behaviours, the more it reinforces the belief that your worth is dependent on others' approval. This can lead to a constant feeling of being 'less than' or not good enough, which in turn drives more people-pleasing behaviour.

But your worth is not dependent on the opinions or approval of others. Your worth is inherent. It's not something that can be earned or lost. It's not dependent on how much you do for others, how much you achieve or how much others like you. You are worthy simply because you exist. Breaking free from the people-pleasing cycle necessitates building a sense of self-worth that is independent of others' opinions, challenging and changing negative self-beliefs, practising self-compassion, and learning to validate and affirm yourself.

When people stop being pleased

Prepare yourself for a dose of reality: when you make the courageous decision to stop people-pleasing, you'll encounter varied reactions from those around you. The truth is, when you shift from constantly accommodating others to prioritising your own needs and boundaries, it will come as a surprise to those who have grown accustomed to your accommodating nature and some people won't like it.

In some cases, though, you'll find that people respect you more when you stop people-pleasing. By asserting your boundaries and standing up for yourself, you demonstrate a newfound strength and self-assuredness that can earn admiration from others. They may appreciate your authenticity and admire your ability to prioritise your own well-being.

Some will be appalled by your change in behaviour, because when you stop people-pleasing, people will stop being pleased with you. This reaction is especially likely if your relationship with them has been built upon a foundation of one-sided (or two-sided) people-pleasing or if people-pleasing is deeply ingrained within your family or cultural dynamics. They may struggle to comprehend or accept your new way of being as it challenges the familiar roles and expectations they have come to rely upon.

Their reactions aren't a reflection of your worth or value. The discomfort they experience is often a result of their own attachment to the dynamics of people-pleasing. It can be challenging to witness their disappointment or disapproval, which is why it's important to build your self-worth alongside unwinding people-pleasing. While the reactions of others may vary, staying true to yourself will lead you towards more fulfilling and balanced relationships based on mutual respect and genuine connection.

Client Story

Respect from others is exactly what my client Holly has experienced as she's worked on reducing people-pleasing: 'I have built my self-love and value in how I show up for myself and the decisions I choose to make in life. With confidence and by increasing my self-esteem, I have shown up to others more authentically, even when that goes against the herd. I try to be aware when I am acting for someone else's gain or if I am seeking approval of my own self-worth. This is an ongoing skill that gets stronger and stronger every time I put it into practice. My friends and even new people I meet notice my self-authenticity and I have found I receive a lot of respect and admiration from staying true to myself. When others have been upset by the choices I make, I am now quick to cognitively realise it is their own stuff which they are presenting and has nothing really to do with me – I am not responsible for other people's thoughts and emotions about me.'

Although it may be a huge shift for you to do things this way, remember, though, that doesn't mean others will even notice, as my client Charlotte was surprised to find: *There were some challenging reactions, but some reactions were surprisingly neutral, just, "Okay, fine!" I was surprised how easy it was.*

Planting Seeds of Authenticity

In the garden of your mind, there stands a majestic oak tree. Its branches stretch wide and its roots are deeply embedded in the fertile soil. This oak tree represents the automatic thoughts and behaviours that have established themselves over time, shaping your people-pleasing tendencies. It's grown tall and mighty, providing shade and shelter, but it also casts a shadow over your authentic self.

Nestled somewhere else in your garden is a delicate sapling. This sapling represents the new thoughts and behaviours that challenge the status quo. It's a tender shoot, requiring care and attention to grow and flourish. And it's important that it receives it, because these emerging thoughts and behaviours will redefine your sense of self-worth, free you from the people-pleasing cycle, and allow you to embrace your true desires and needs.

Nurturing this sapling requires intentional effort. Just as you would water and protect a young plant, you must tend to these new thoughts and behaviours, starting with recognising that the automatic thoughts, represented by the towering oak tree, have dominated your landscape for far too long. They may have served a purpose in the past, but now they're holding you back.

To cultivate the new sapling, you must challenge the deep-rooted beliefs and patterns associated with people-pleasing by gently questioning the thoughts and behaviours that stem from the oak tree: Are they aligned with your authentic self? Do they honour your needs and desires? Allow the young sapling to root down and take hold by consciously nurturing and reinforcing the new thoughts and behaviours that help you to express what you really want to say.

Just as the sapling needs sunlight to grow, seek out supportive environments and relationships that encourage your personal growth. Surround yourself with individuals who value your authentic self and respect your boundaries. Engage in self-compassion and self-acceptance, recognising that unwinding established automatic thoughts takes time and patience. With each small victory, the new thoughts and behaviours gain strength and become more ingrained.

Stepping out of the protective shade of the oak tree requires courage. It means challenging the familiar and venturing into the unknown. It may feel uncomfortable at first, as if you're leaving behind the security of what you've always known. But as you do it, you'll start to realise that the shade of the oak tree wasn't as protective as it seemed. In fact, it may have kept you from fully experiencing the warmth of the sun and the vast expanse of possibilities that lie beyond. You'll come to understand that you don't need the shade of the oak tree, because your inner strength and self-worth are more than enough to guide you on your journey.

With time, nourishment and support, the sapling will grow, eventually overshadowing the oak tree, taking its place as the dominant force in your mental landscape. The more you consciously nurture the growth of new thoughts and behaviours, the more they will thrive and replace the outdated patterns that no longer serve you. With time, the sapling will flourish, guiding you towards a life where your worth is not defined by the approval of others, but rather by your own self-acceptance and self-love. By unwinding people-pleasing behaviours, you will free yourself up to be yourself. With that comes intimacy, trust and generosity – and you'll help others simply because you want to.

Chapter 6

Emotions

'You're so emotional' is thrown about as an insult. Ironically, it's usually the person issuing the insult who's emotional, but it's far more comfortable to put it on someone else than accept the reality of what's going on inside us. I've been told I am emotional myself on many, many occasions and it used to really bother me. Most of the time it was by men who were trying to dismiss or provoke me, but there have been women who've said it to me too – I suspect because of the sexist stereotypes and beliefs that we've all unconsciously absorbed.

In fact, it was my own internalised patriarchy that had me believing being emotional was bad and something to be avoided at all costs or at least kept hidden. That was because, in my young brain, being emotional equated to being female and being female meant being less than – and nobody wants to be less than. So instead I sided with the patriarchal belief that women are emotional, and therefore unreliable and untrustworthy. I probably told other women – in my head or out loud – that they were too emotional. Ugh. Patriarchy really has done a number on us.

These days, on the rare occasion that someone dares to suggest that I'm being emotional, it doesn't get my back up at all, because regardless of whether their opinion is correct or not, I accept it as the truth: I *am* emotional. Being emotional is part of the human experience and that's not a problem for me. It's something I choose to celebrate, so even when it's offered as an insult, I receive it as a compliment, which tends to confuse the hell out of the other person.

Anyway, the notion of trying to eradicate our emotions is not only unrealistic, but also unwise. Emotions are an inherent part of our human experience and attempting to suppress or eliminate them would be counterproductive. Rather than viewing emotions as a problem to be solved, recognise the immense benefits they bring to our lives, serving as an internal compass, guiding us towards what matters, and providing valuable insights into our needs, desires and values. We are all emotional. That's not the problem. The problem is that we don't know *how* to be emotional.

You Are Not an Emotion

Whether you feel excited or anxious, remember that those words describe how you *feel*, not who you *are*. There's a big difference between 'I'm anxious' and 'I feel anxious' – test them out and see how they both feel. 'I'm anxious' has a sense of permanence to it – the anxiety is part of who I am, whereas 'I feel anxious' acknowledges that I do feel anxious and at the same time also creates space to transition into feeling something else. This distinction is crucial, because it reminds us that emotions are transient; they come and go. Your current emotional state is temporary and not a permanent part of your identity.

I've met plenty of people who, when describing themselves say, 'I'm an anxious person' and, while that is true – they are prone to experiencing anxiety – the more they say that, the more that neural groove deepens and it becomes part of their identity.

Similarly, someone might say, 'I'm depressed,' because they have a medical diagnosis of depression, but we don't do that for other diagnoses. Nobody says 'I'm chicken pox' or 'I'm arthritic.' The power of language is immense; it's not just a tool for communication, but also a powerful shaper of our thoughts and emotions. The words we use to describe our feelings can influence how we perceive and experience those feelings. So, I recommend that you keep the 'feeling' when you're describing how you feel. By being mindful of our language, we can gain more control over our emotional experiences.

A Disturbance in the Force

Emotions are complex and multifaceted phenomena that play a crucial role in our lives. Like waves on the ocean of our lives, they rise and fall, and ebb and flow, in response to the world within us and around us. Each of us experiences these waves differently, depending on what rocks our boat, and so specific responses and intensity can vary greatly from individual to individual.

Your emotions are real and valid, but it's important to remember that they're not the gospel truth. They're not facts, but rather your personal, subjective responses to yourself and the world around you. Emotions are somatic – or bodily – patterns of response. They convey valuable information about our internal and external world. These changes in the body often drive expression and movement. All emotions require energy, they are 'expensive' in that sense, but the body is willing to pay this cost, because of the benefits we derive from them.

Emotions are fluid and naturally change or evolve into other emotions or into a place of resolution. If we don't move past intense emotions like anger, fear and joy, we risk running the body at a high cost, which can lead to problems and create more intense feelings and thinking patterns. Instead, we can aim to return to a baseline state, much like a thermostat resetting itself.

Client Story

At the simplest level, emotions come as they come, delivering their message and value. They help us become emotionally competent and teach us about ourselves and the world around us, as my client Zoe describes:

'I realised I had been racing through life not noticing or feeling my feelings. Therefore, I was overwhelmed and stressed, and using food to stuff the emotions down. I was also snapping at my partner a lot and not getting the best from myself at work, but now I realise that I'd never been taught about my nervous system and emotions, so uncovering all this required some support. The power of accepting that "whatever you're feeling is okay!" has been hugely helpful. Understanding emotions and how to process them safely has been so useful. I have kind words to say to myself. I regularly check in with how I'm feeling and address my needs. I have set boundaries and improved my relationships because of them.'

However, when we add personal history and stories to the mix, understanding emotions can become more complicated. It's like stirring a spoonful of complexity into our emotional soup. No matter how complex it gets, though, it all shows up in the body. We can move through this, let go and come back to a state of balance. After all, who hasn't felt better after a good cry?

Emotions, Feelings and Moods

Emotions, feelings and moods, while interconnected, are distinct phenomena that play crucial roles in our lives. Emotions originate as sensations in the body that can be experienced consciously and subconsciously as immediate responses to stimuli. They are brief, lasting anywhere from seconds to minutes. When you receive a text from someone and their name pops up on your screen, you probably react by experiencing an immediate emotion of some kind – perhaps joy, surprise or anxiety. Emotions can be thought of as raw data, the body's initial, unfiltered response to an event, but as soon as you start to frame your emotional response, you experience feelings.

Feelings, on the other hand, are the conscious interpretation of these emotions. They are generated by your thoughts and are experienced consciously. When you saw that text, you had an emotional response, which you then used your thoughts to identify and make sense of. This is where feelings come into play. For example, the physical sensations of a racing heart and sweaty palms could be interpreted as either anxiety or excitement, depending on the context and your thoughts about the situation. Unlike the clear-cut nature of emotions, feelings are subject to interpretation and the narrative you tell yourself.

Moods are longer-lasting states that can persist for hours or even days. If they extend into weeks or years, they might be classified as mood disorders. Moods can be thought of as states of mind that influence how you think and behave. Unlike emotions, which are typically responses to specific events, moods don't necessarily depend on a particular trigger. They can be influenced by a variety of factors, including physical health, exposure to light, diet, physical activity and your thought patterns. Moods are more about how you feel over a sustained period.

So in summary, motions are the body's immediate responses, feelings are our conscious interpretation of these responses, and moods are longer-lasting states that influence our thinking and behaviour.

More Than a Feeling

Experiencing an emotion begins with a spark, a trigger that sets off a cascade of reactions in your body and mind. First, your neurophysiology is aroused. This is like the opening beat of a song, setting the rhythm for what's to come.

Your heart rate might increase, your palms might sweat and you might feel a flutter in your stomach. These physiological changes are your body's way of preparing for action.

Next, your motor behaviour is influenced. This is the dance itself; the visible expression of your emotion. It could be as subtle as a change in your facial expression, a shift in your posture or a change in your breathing. Or it could be more dramatic and explicit, such as running away from a threat or reaching out for a hug.

Finally, you enter a subjective feeling state that can bias your behaviour. This is the emotional high note; the crescendo of the song. It's the feeling of fear that makes you avoid dark alleys or the feeling of joy that makes you laugh out loud. This subjective feeling state is what gives each emotion its unique flavour and guides your behaviour accordingly. Every time you experience an emotion, you're experiencing way more than a feeling – it's a complex dance of physiological arousal, physical movement and subjective experience.

The Power and Purpose of Emotions

Emotions might not always be comfortable, but they're always valuable. Take fear and anger, for instance. They're intense, they're disruptive and they can be downright uncomfortable. But they need to be, because they're central to our survival. They're like the alarm system of our body, alerting us to potential threats and mobilising us to take action.

When we encounter an object, creature, person or situation, our emotions spring into action. They capture our attention, influence our perception and shape our memories. For instance, think back to a meeting with your boss. Your emotions during that meeting didn't just colour your experience, they also influenced how you remembered it.

Emotions also play a starring role in our relationships with ourselves and others. They're the glue that binds us together, facilitating the development and maintenance of social bonds, and helping us to understand one another. Displays of emotion allow us to guess how others are feeling, but we're not always accurate in our assumptions. If someone is crying, you might conclude that they feel sad. However, if they told you that they're pregnant after years of fertility issues, then their tears would take on a whole new meaning and you would likely interpret their tears as ones of joy.

You might not always love the experience of your emotions, but that doesn't stop them from being valuable. They are central to our everyday human experience, so instead of treating them as intruders, see them as guides, messengers and storytellers (just remember to question what they're saying).

Safety Dance

Emotions play a crucial role in our memory and behaviour. They act like highlighters, marking important experiences in our minds so that we remember them vividly. This is because emotionally charged events activate the amygdala, the part of the brain that's involved in emotional processing and memory formation. When you encounter a situation that triggers a strong emotion, your brain takes note and stores it for future reference. This is why we tend to remember emotionally charged events, like a surprise birthday party or a scary movie, more vividly than everyday occurrences.

Emotions also choreograph your behaviour to keep you safe. For instance, fear can prompt us to avoid potentially dangerous situations, while disgust can steer us away from things that might make us sick. This is an adaptive response that has helped us survive as a species. In other words, it's a very good thing, but emotions can also bias our thoughts and memories. Research has shown that our current emotional state can colour our memories of past events. If you're feeling happy, you're more likely to recall positive memories, while if you're feeling sad, you might remember more negative events. This is known as mood-congruent memory.

Shiny, Happy People Laughing

Labelling emotions as either positive or negative, while convenient for casual conversation, can be misleading and even harmful. By categorising emotions in this way, we risk creating a mindset where so-called negative emotions are seen as undesirable and something to be avoided. Add to this the fact that so-called negative emotions don't feel great and it's easy to end up in a situation where you fear your own emotions, while also judging yourself for having them in the first place.

This perspective is further reinforced by the prevalence of happy, celebratory images on social media, which can create the illusion that everyone else is constantly happy. But let's be real – this obsession with happiness is overrated.

Client Story

Expecting to be happy all the time is a surefire recipe for disappointment, as my client Laura found: 'I was never taught or modelled how to deal with my emotions or create safety for myself so, of course, I didn't know how. I thought I was meant to be more or less happy all the time and because I wasn't that meant I was doing life wrong. But now I know that all emotions are part of life and I can practise feeling all my emotions, even the hard ones. I can love myself and have compassion for myself in good and bad times. And that I have so much agency in my life and nothing is set in stone. And I don't have to settle.

'This really helped with the feelings of frustration; that I can feel it and let it be there, and change things. I used to often feel trapped or limited based on past decisions. I think feeling my feelings, actually really loving and accepting myself, and seeing all the amazing things and changes that members do and make in the community, have helped me indefinitely. I still experience really strong emotions that are sometimes difficult for me and I want to get answers as to why I'm feeling them, but now it's with curiosity and compassion instead of fear and overwhelm. I can better name when I'm feeling lonely or sad or frustrated, and regulate myself afterwards and express my needs. In general, I now trust myself that whatever I feel, I'll always manage to get back to feeling me again and that trust feels amazing.'

Instead of putting all your emotional eggs in the happiness basket, I recommend embracing the full spectrum of your emotions. By doing so, you'll discover the unique value that each emotion holds and the overall value of being an emotional being. Emotions, even those often labelled as negative, can provide valuable information, motivate us to take action and help us connect with others.

Don't fret – I'm not suggesting you dive headfirst into the deep end without a life jacket. We'll explore these more challenging emotions together and I'll share some of my favourite techniques for experiencing them. Remember, all emotions, whether joy or sorrow, excitement or fear, have their place in our emotional landscape. By embracing them all, we can live a richer, more authentic life.

The dark side of unrelenting optimism

In today's era of inspirational quotes, endless Instagram stories and motivational memes, the pressure to be positive can seem omnipresent. Just think positive! Everything happens for a reason! At first glance, positivity seems like a desirable trait. After all, who wouldn't want to lead a life full of optimism, hope and joy? However, it can morph into *toxic positivity* when it's forced, rather than genuinely felt.

Toxic positivity refers to the overzealous application of happiness and optimism, even when situations are grave. Instead of offering solace, it suppresses authentic feelings, leading to increased stress, anxiety and a feeling of isolation. By constantly painting over authentic emotions with positivity, we deny ourselves the experience of the full range of human emotions and all they have to offer, losing opportunities for genuine insight and understanding.

Positive Thinking Pressures When Trying to Conceive

Many of my clients who are trying to conceive express a daunting obligation to remain endlessly positive. Undergoing fertility treatments places individuals in what I'd describe as a 'hormonally vulnerable' phase. These treatments involve taking hormones at a level that far surpasses what the body would typically produce and reactions to them can be full-on, emotionally and physically.

Assisted reproductive processes also bear their own set of pressures. Not only is it an intense physiological and psychological journey, but it also comes with significant financial implications. For some, it may be the only treatment cycle they can access through their NHS trust or finance privately. Then there are the other emotional strains that come with the territory of a fertility journey. It's no surprise, then, that it feels like a high-stakes situation and the flood of advice from various quarters about the need to stay optimistic only adds to the stress.

The tendency to gravitate towards controlling one aspect – our mindset – when so much is beyond our control, is only human, but the brain is hardwired to anticipate potential hazards. This inclination towards cautiousness has been pivotal in our evolution, allowing us to learn from past pain and trauma. However, in the context of fertility treatments this innate tendency can backfire.

I've witnessed clients berate themselves for not maintaining an impossibly upbeat outlook, as if one's positivity could be precisely measured and calibrated to sustain human life. They internalise any negative thought, interpreting it as a personal failure. Should a treatment cycle not result in pregnancy, they blame their inability to 'stay positive'. Yet expecting anyone – especially those navigating the tumultuous waters of assisted reproduction – to exist in a perpetual state of unblemished optimism is unrealistic and, sadly, the emotions of guilt, self-doubt and perceived failure, layered on top of the already-present challenges, only compound the weight of the journey.

Our brains are not engineered to function as relentless optimism machines. By nature, they're vigilantly scanning for potential threats. Expecting constant positivity amid such a profound journey is not only unrealistic, it's counterintuitive.

Client Story

Over the past couple of years Ann has been on a long fertility journey that's been littered with recurring heartbreak and disappointment. She describes it as losing touch with herself: 'Everything felt as if I was seeing through a dense fog; kind of subdued; like a wet blanket had spread over me. I knew there were things in my life I could be grateful for, that bring me joy, yet somehow I felt so low that I couldn't truly bathe in the joyfulness. I wanted to, but I couldn't. This left me feeling stuck and it became harder and harder to go into the next fertility treatment cycle with an open heart and soul.

'I am usually a resilient and optimistic person. However, these kinds of experiences completely drained me and I didn't have the tools to rebuild my resilience. I was keeping a brave face and soldiered on when internally I would curse the world. I didn't want to burden anyone with my struggles, so what I now know to be toxic positivity (see page 114) was my go-to.

'Detecting and understanding my subconscious thought patterns was an absolute game-changer. To start there and then learn about my nervous system really helped me pause, take a step back and look at what's going on in my head. This consequently led to more self-compassion, which was such a marvellous thing to acquire!

'I've also learned to own my emotions. Of course, I was feeling like shit when another cycle failed and another embryo didn't implant. This helped me shift my focus so that my fertility journey wasn't this all-encompassing thing dominating my life. I found my way back to my centred and grounded self. I started thinking about other things that might be cool for me to pursue in my future. I even came to terms with potentially staying child-free and I really was okay with that. And then, suddenly, I was pregnant. Without help from doctors and nurses! The work I did in the past year with Maisie helped clear my head, shift my focus and eventually free me up. Which is amazing! I've become even more patient than I've already been (with regards to other people), while simultaneously staying present and mindful of my own needs and emotions.'

Ann's experience underscores the importance of not masking our struggles underneath a veneer of unwavering positivity. Embracing the full spectrum of our emotions, seeking understanding and having self-compassion are far kinder and more useful. In a world that often peddles the notion of positivity at all costs, it's important to cultivate spaces where genuine emotions are honoured and holistic well-being is championed.

Emotional Echoes

Emotions are shaped by our interactions with others, especially during our formative years. This is where emotional modelling comes into play. Emotional modelling refers to the process by which we learn to understand and express our emotions by observing others, particularly our parents, caregivers and peers. For instance, a child might learn to express anger by observing how their parents express this emotion.

However, the way these significant figures respond to our emotions can also have a profound impact. If a child is mocked for crying when they feel upset, they might learn to suppress their sadness. If anger is more acceptable, they might learn to express their upset through anger. Whereas if someone was sent to their room for expressing anger, they might learn to associate anger with isolation and repress it. If excitement is frowned upon, they might learn to dampen their joy.

These early experiences can shape our emotional landscape in profound ways, influencing how we express and regulate our emotions in adulthood. They can also impact our emotional intelligence – our ability to understand, use and manage our emotions in beneficial ways. So, the next time you find yourself reacting to an emotion in a certain way, take a moment to reflect. Consider the emotional programming you received growing up, how that might be influencing your emotional dance today and whether you want to unwind any aspect of how you were raised.

Common Emotions

Some emotions will feel more do-able to you than others, but let's take a closer look at some of the more charged and challenging ones.

Loneliness

Loneliness sucks. It's no wonder that so many of us will do anything we can to avoid feeling it – drinking alcohol, endlessly scrolling on our phones, having unsatisfying sex in a bid to feel connection, and hanging out in groups of people that aren't a match for our values and desires are all examples of how we do this.

Loneliness is a complex emotional response to isolation or lack of companionship. It can be triggered by a variety of situations, from physical isolation to feeling misunderstood or disconnected from others. You can spend plenty of time around other people and still experience loneliness, just as someone can spend plenty of time alone and not feel lonely.

Loneliness can be particularly challenging to feel, because it often comes with a sense of longing and unfulfilled social needs, and chronic loneliness can have serious health implications, including increased risk of cardiovascular disease, depression and cognitive decline. But while loneliness is a painful emotion, its *prosocial value* lies in its ability to motivate us to seek social connections and form bonds with others. It can drive us to reach out, communicate and engage in social activities.

Positive Social Relations

Prosocial refers to thoughts, feelings or behaviours that are intended to help or benefit others. It includes things like helping, sharing, donating, cooperating and volunteering. Prosocial emotions are specific feelings that motivate individuals to act in ways that benefit others or promote positive social relations. These emotions are integral to fostering cooperation, maintaining social bonds and building cohesive communities. Some prosocial emotions and their related actions include:

- Empathy: When we empathise – or feel and understand what another person is experiencing – we're more likely to offer help, comfort or support, because we can put ourselves in their shoes.
- Compassion: This deep feeling of concern for someone who is suffering, coupled with a desire to alleviate their pain, can lead to acts of kindness or charity.
- Gratitude: Recognising and appreciating the positive actions of others, and expressing gratitude, can foster positive relationships and people who feel grateful are often more likely to 'pay it forward.'

The existence of prosocial emotions suggests that humans have evolved to live in social groups and that these feelings play a fundamental role in maintaining group cohesion and cooperation. Prosocial emotions drive prosocial behaviours, reinforcing the bonds that hold societies together and promoting the well-being of its community.

Fear

Fear is a basic survival mechanism that alerts us to the presence of danger, activating the stress response system. Fear can be experienced as a rapid heartbeat, quickened breath and heightened alertness. While fear can be protective, it can also be challenging when it becomes chronic or disproportionate to the situation, as seen in phobias and anxiety disorders. Fear can promote prosocial behaviour by motivating protective actions not only for oneself, but also for others in one's social group, such as warning them of a potential danger.

Anxiety

Anxiety is a feeling of unease that can be mild or severe. It's a normal and often healthy emotion that can be helpful, because of its ability to make you more aware and responsive, thus improving your performance. However, regularly feeling disproportionate levels of anxiety can be related to anxiety disorders that lead to excessive nervousness, fear, apprehension and worry. These disorders alter how a person processes emotions and behaves, also causing physical symptoms. Similar to fear, anxiety can lead to prosocial behaviours by encouraging individuals to seek support from others. It can also make people more attuned to threats in their environment, leading them to take actions that protect their social group.

Guilt

Guilt is a moral emotion that occurs when a person believes they have violated a moral standard and bears the responsibility for that violation. It's a deeply personal emotion that is often tied to our conscience or moral compass. For many of my clients, it's a difficult emotion to process, because it involves a critical evaluation of one's actions and can lead to feelings of shame and unworthiness. Guilt is a highly prosocial emotion. It often arises when we believe we have done something wrong that has harmed others. The feeling of guilt can motivate reparative behaviours, such as apologies, making amends, or engaging in behaviour that benefits the person who was harmed.

Shame

Shame is a painful emotion that stems from a negative evaluation of the self. It involves feelings of worthlessness, embarrassment and humiliation. Shame can be particularly challenging to feel, because it strikes at the core of our identity, often leading to a desire to hide or escape. It has long been said that shame has prosocial effects because it can deter individuals from engaging in harmful behaviours that could damage their social relationships or social standing, and motivating them to make amends after a wrong-doing.

However, others argue that it can also have significant negative effects, such as:

- Internalisation and lowered self-esteem: Shame often involves a negative evaluation of the self, which can lead to feelings of worthlessness and damage to self-esteem. This internalisation of shame can contribute to mental health issues, including depression and anxiety.
- Avoidance and withdrawal: Rather than motivating prosocial behaviour, shame can lead individuals to avoid the situation or people involved in an attempt to escape the painful feelings. This avoidance can harm relationships, careers and lead to social isolation.
- Aggression and antisocial behaviour: Some research suggests that shame can contribute to aggression and antisocial behaviour. This is particularly the case when individuals externalise their shame by blaming others for their negative feelings, leading to anger and hostility instead of prosocial behaviours.
- Shame versus guilt: Some psychologists differentiate between shame and guilt in terms of their prosocial value. They suggest that while guilt (a recognition that one's actions were wrong) can motivate reparative behaviour, shame (a negative evaluation of the self) is more likely to lead to avoidance, withdrawal or aggression.

While shame can sometimes have prosocial outcomes, it is also associated with significant negative effects. The impact of shame can depend on a variety of factors, including how it is managed, the individual's psychological resilience, and their social and cultural context.

Client Story

My client Stephanie eloquently describes the healing power of community: 'Living in an activated nervous system state – either in fight, flight, freeze or please-and-appease – was taking its toll on my energy levels, my engagement with life and affecting my relationships. A difficult childhood had set the scene for ongoing nervous system dysregulation. While I had done some therapy and some trauma work, I was still finding myself stuck in the same old familiar patterns.

'Through being in true community with others, where I have been able to truly be myself and share my darkest and most challenging stuff, I have been able to be seen, heard and celebrated. I have learnt that where I thought there was shame, there was inspiration to others, and the things I hid were actually struggles that others could relate to. By being brave and opening up, getting coached and sharing my self-coaching, I've completely changed my self-concept and how I see myself. Being in a group of people all working through stuff has shown me how normal all the challenges are that I thought were shameful and had to be hidden. I now prioritise caring for my nervous system. I am able to quickly recognise if I'm getting dysregulated and I usually know what to do to get back to a regulated place.'

Anger

Anger is a natural emotion, but it's probably the one my clients struggle with the most. The anger is there, but it's repressed, disguised as frustration and resentment, and buried under the weight of internalised societal beliefs that it's not acceptable for a woman to be angry. Combine that with the strong physical activation that anger causes in the body, such as a racing heartbeat, a tightness in your chest and tense muscles, and it's no wonder that it can feel scary. Anger can have prosocial effects, though, by motivating individuals to confront injustices or stand up for others who are being treated unfairly, driving us to engage in social change or advocate for others.

Anger feels strong and it ought to, because its purpose is to get us to do something. Anger allows us to express negative feelings or react to perceived threats or injustices, but if you haven't had healthy expressions of anger modelled to you, then it makes sense that it feels so challenging to experience. If anger feels dangerous then it could feel safer to keep the lid on and control every word, facial expression and gesture. It's often the premenstrual phase of the cycle that affords us an opportunity to access our anger – a pocket of time where all that's kept down is able to come up. Learning how to access anger is transformative. However, when not managed properly, it can lead to stress, relationship problems and even health issues.

Joy

Joy is experienced in response to something pleasing or satisfying. It's often associated with a sense of contentment, happiness or fulfilment. The beauty of joy lies in its spontaneity and authenticity, but, while joy is generally considered a desirable emotion, it can be challenging for some people to fully experience. Societal expectations, past traumas or self-imposed barriers can hinder the free expression and experience of this emotion.

My client Stephanie illustrates this beautifully: *'It has been and still is challenging for me to experience joy. The commentary in my mind can interfere with experiencing joy – wondering if I'm enjoying something enough or why I don't enjoy something when others do. An over-focus on time can also impact my experience of joy. For example, during a massage, I might spend much of the session wondering how much time is left and feeling sad that it will soon be over.'* This shows that our thoughts can sometimes overpower the present moment, inhibiting the purity of the joy we could be feeling.

For some, guilt swiftly follows and drowns out joy, as Charlotte shared, *'I doubt if I did enough to deserve joy, but the main challenge is that if others suffer in general (which has no relation at all: their suffering and my pleasure) or don't enjoy things, I have thoughts like "You can't enjoy this while others suffer" and "Only if everyone is happy you can feel joy".'* This internal moral compass, while rooted in empathy, can paradoxically rob us of moments of joy.

The barriers to joy can also be tied to past traumas and life experiences. As my client Lizzie describes, *'It was a knee-jerk response to health issues and associated mental health difficulties and life upheavals. Whenever I felt joy from the age of 13 to 21, my immediate thought was "This won't last" and then I felt afraid again. It was like I didn't want to know what I was missing the next "inevitable" time it all went wrong. I also didn't have a great understanding of what brought me joy: I'm autistic and I very rarely get it socially. I didn't realise I could create my own joy and I didn't know how to.'* Lizzie's candid reflection illustrates that joy can sometimes be a foreign or fleeting concept due to past hardships, as well as highlighting that joy doesn't have a one-size-fits-all definition. It's a deeply personal emotion, and the way we experience it will vary depending on our personal histories, neurological differences and life circumstances.

Jealousy

Jealousy is a complex emotion that often involves feelings of insecurity, fear and anxiety over an anticipated loss of something of great personal value, particularly in reference to a human connection. It often consists of a combination of emotions such as anger, resentment, inadequacy, helplessness and disgust. While jealousy is often seen as a negative emotion, it can motivate us to make changes and improve matters, such as contributing more to relationships or engaging in behaviours that improve our social standing.

Humiliation

Humiliation can be felt when someone loses self-respect or dignity. It's often associated with feelings of shame and embarrassment. Humiliation is particularly challenging to feel, because it involves a sense of being lowered or degraded, but it can also deter individuals from repeating behaviours that led to their humiliation, potentially steering them away from antisocial or harmful behaviours.

Hopelessness

Hopelessness is characterised by a bleak outlook on the future. It involves feelings of despair and a loss of optimism or belief in positive outcomes. Hopelessness can be particularly challenging to feel, because it can lead to feelings of apathy and resignation, and is often associated with depression. While hopelessness is a difficult emotion, when shared, it can foster empathy and support from others, leading to prosocial behaviours such as providing comfort or assistance.

That's all very well in theory, but the challenge comes in being able to reach out to others when you're feeling this way, especially if you're prone to putting yourself down for being able to do so. This is where being aware of your stress responses is essential. Remember that the freeze response can feel like a collapse or shutdown of the system and a loss of connection – from yourself, others and your environment – which means it can feel infinitely harder to reach out to others for help. That's because it *is* harder.

Emotional Highways

Ingrained habits around certain emotions form through a process known as emotional habituation. This process is deeply rooted in the brain's reward system and is influenced by repeated exposure to specific emotional stimuli, like a favourite song or the scent of a hospital, or internal stimuli, such as thoughts and the recollection of memories.

When we repeatedly experience a certain emotion in response to a specific situation, our brain begins to form a neural pathway associated with that emotion. Each time the situation is encountered and the emotion is experienced, this pathway is reinforced. Over time, the pathway becomes so well-trodden that the emotional response becomes automatic, forming an ingrained emotional habit, as is the case with the Sunday Scaries – when some people feel anxious or sad on Sunday evenings, dreading the upcoming working week. Even if they enjoy their job, the repeated emotional response of anxiety as Sunday night approaches can become a habit. With time, the mere realisation that it's Sunday evening, even without any explicit thought about work, can trigger feelings of unease. This emotional response is a result of the brain having reinforced the association between Sunday evenings and the emotion of anxiety or dread. This process is a fundamental principle of neuroplasticity, which is the brain's ability to reorganise itself by forming new neural connections throughout life.

What Fires Together Wires Together

There is a principle known as Hebb's rule, which states that when neurons fire at the same time, the connections between them strengthen. Over time, these strengthened connections can form new neural pathways. When first learning to play the guitar, every chord and note requires conscious thought and deliberate finger placement. So. Much. Concentration. The brain is making new connections as you try to coordinate your fingers to produce the desired sound. The neurons involved in the process are 'firing together.'

As you practise, the same sets of neurons continue to fire in sequence. With time and consistent practice, the connections between these neurons strengthen, the act of playing a chord becomes more fluid and you no longer have to think consciously about each finger's placement. The sequences of neurons have 'wired together' through repetition.

This neural reinforcement through repetition is why, after enough practice, playing the guitar (or any other learned skill) becomes almost second nature. The brain has optimised the neural pathway for this activity due to the repeated firing of the same sequence of neurons. The more frequently a specific pattern of neurons is activated (due to repeated experiences or practice), the stronger the connections between those neurons become. This foundational concept is the basis for many learning and memory processes in the brain.

The principle of 'what fires together wires together' applies to emotional stimuli just as it does to motor or cognitive skills. Your brain doesn't just form connections in response to actions or thought patterns; it also forms connections in response to emotional experiences.

Let's say every time a child is presented with a particular stimulus, like a loud noise, they simultaneously experience a negative emotion, like fear. Over time, just the anticipation of the loud noise, or even something that reminds the child of it, might trigger the emotion of fear. The neurons representing the loud noise and the emotion of fear have fired together so frequently that they've 'wired together'. This is a basic form of associative learning and it's the foundation of classical conditioning, a concept introduced by Russian physiologist Ivan Pavlov. In Pavlov's experiment, dogs were conditioned to associate the sound of a bell with being fed. Eventually, they began to salivate just hearing the bell, even without the presence of food

In cases of trauma, an event elicits a strong emotional response. The context or elements of that traumatic situation – like a specific location, smell or sound – can become associated with the intense emotional response. Later on, encountering a similar context or element can trigger the same emotional response, even if the traumatic event itself isn't happening again. The emotional response and the contextual cues have fired together so powerfully that their association is deeply encoded. This is how emotional habits become ingrained.

Suppose a person experiences anxiety when they have to speak in public. Each time they're asked to give a presentation or speak in a meeting, they feel anxious. In response to this anxiety, they might start avoiding situations where they have to speak publicly – declining invitations to present and staying quiet in meetings. The neurons associated with public speaking and the neurons associated with anxiety are firing together, so over time, a neural pathway linking public speaking and anxiety forms. Then, as the person repeatedly responds to their anxiety by avoiding public speaking altogether, another neural pathway forms, linking anxiety with avoidance behaviours. This creates an ingrained emotional habit: when faced with public speaking, the person feels anxious and then avoids the situation. With time, even the thought of public speaking could trigger this habitual response, due to the strength of the neural pathways that have been formed.

The principle of 'what fires together wires together' helps us to understand how our experiences – including our emotions – shape our brains and our behaviour, forming emotional habits. Don't be put off by the idea of decades-old emotional habits; with conscious effort and consistent practice, it is possible to form new, healthier emotional habits. In this example, the person could practise public speaking in a safe and supportive environment, talking about a topic that they love, which could help them form a new neural pathway linking public speaking with positive emotions. Over time, this could help them break their habit of avoidance and respond to public speaking with confidence instead of anxiety.

Thankfully, the sensory experiences of nervousness and excitement are similar, providing a quick way to shift your experience. Both are emotional states that provoke physiological responses that stem the fight-or-flight response. Both nervousness and excitement can lead to:

- Increased heart rate
- Faster breathing or shortness of breath
- Butterflies in the stomach (a fluttery feeling or stomach churning)
- Sweating
- Feeling jittery or shaky
- Heightened alertness.

These responses arise from the activation of the sympathetic nervous system, which prepares the body for quick action. Both emotions also involve a level of anticipation and focus on a forthcoming event or situation. Whether you're excited about a positive outcome or nervous about a potentially negative one, your mind is directed towards the future. Nervousness and excitement tend to elevate your energy levels, making you feel more awake, alert or even restless.

The difference between them lies more in our interpretation of these physiological signals than the signals themselves and, by focusing on the similarities between nervousness and excitement, it becomes easier to understand how you can reframe one emotion as the other. When it comes to experiences like public speaking:

- Reframe the narrative: If you feel nervous before a public speaking event, acknowledging the physiological symptoms and then consciously reframing them can be helpful. Instead of thinking, 'I'm so nervous,' tell yourself, 'I'm excited about this opportunity to share my thoughts.'
- Embrace the energy: Use the heightened energy to your advantage. If you interpret the extra energy as excitement, it can enhance your presentation, making you more passionate and engaged.
- Mindset shift: Recognising that every time you feel 'nervous' it could just as easily be 'excitement' gives you power over your emotions. This shift in perspective can make the situation feel less intimidating and more like an opportunity.

My client Stephanie played around with this on a family outing: *'I experimented with the feelings of fear and excitement when I went to a forest high ropes course with my husband. I realised that the feelings in my body were very similar and also that they are just feelings, so I could play around with them and play with how I named them. I also realised that the sensations didn't have to hold me back and I could take the leap (literally) even if I was feeling fear.'*

By consciously choosing to interpret your body's signals as excitement rather than nervousness, you can approach challenges like public speaking with a more positive and confident mindset. This doesn't mean ignoring genuine concerns or underestimating the importance of preparation, but it's about harnessing the energy your body is providing in a way that serves you better.

The Journey Towards Emotional Proficiency

Building emotional proficiency is a lot like learning a new language – the language of your body and emotions. In doing so, you'll become fluent in understanding and interpreting the signals your body sends you, and responding to them in a constructive way. Emotional proficiency involves several key skills, each separate but related:

Recognition

Learning to identify the emotions you're experiencing is like learning the vocabulary of a new language. Each emotion has its own unique 'signature' in your body; a specific set of physical sensations and changes.

Interpretation

Once you've identified an emotion, the next step is to understand what it's trying to tell you. This is like making sense of the words or translating a sentence from another language, with each emotion carrying a message about your needs, desires or boundaries. Sometimes you might immediately understand its message or it may take time and only hit you later on.

Response

Finally, emotional proficiency involves knowing how to respond to your emotions in a way that serves your well-being. This is like carrying on a conversation and being able to influence the direction that it goes in, both listening and taking part. It's about engaging with your emotions, rather than ignoring or suppressing them.

Emotional vocabulary

As you become more proficient in recognising and interpreting your emotions, you'll also start to develop a richer and more nuanced emotional vocabulary. Think about it as expanding your vocabulary in a new language. You'll move beyond basic labels like happy or sad, and start to use more specific words like elated, content, melancholic or despondent. Having a rich emotional vocabulary not only allows you to describe your feelings more accurately, but also helps you to understand and respond to them more effectively. It's the difference between knowing you're feeling bad and understanding that you're feeling frustrated, lonely or disappointed. Each of these emotions has different implications and might require different responses, so being able to distinguish between them is a key part of emotional proficiency.

Client Story

Sarah felt unable to take risks or jump in feet first without looking. She was harbouring a lot of anger, which was affecting her relationships, and she was very hard on herself. Sarah was carrying some very old thought patterns around and, combined with the confronting impact of perimenopause, she knew it was time to look at them, because she was feeling knackered, stuck and ground down.

By focusing on experiencing her emotions, Sarah is creating a new relationship with herself. She says, 'The main thing for me at the moment is allowing myself to feel the feelings – to welcome them in. This is really hard at times and I sometimes just look at them from the sidelines and don't open the door to them, but when I do, I realise it's not so scary and there's so much I can learn from just sitting and letting my emotions be. Previously I would have stuffed them down with food, but this got me nowhere. I'm starting to accept myself exactly as I am.'

Remember, it's okay to be a beginner in this process and there's no such thing as getting it wrong. You might find that some emotions are easier for you to handle than others, probably the ones that were more acceptable to your caregivers and peers growing up, but that's perfectly normal.

A word of warning, though: as you become more proficient at feeling your emotions, you may find that you're feeling more than before. This might seem overwhelming and your brain might tell you that something's gone wrong, especially if you're used to avoiding your emotions. But remember, these emotions are already there. By becoming more proficient at feeling them, you're not creating new emotions, you're simply becoming more aware of what's already there. Building emotional proficiency is a journey, not a destination. It's a lifelong process of learning, growth and self-discovery.

Broad Strokes to Fine Details

Learning to identify your emotions is like learning to read a map of your internal landscape. At first, the terrain might seem unfamiliar and confusing, but with practice, you'll start to recognise landmarks and navigate with ease.

When you're first starting out, go with what's obvious to you. Psychologists often refer to the broader categories as the 'basic' emotions, which include happiness, sadness, fear, anger, surprise and disgust.

Once you've come up with the broad category of emotion you're experiencing, you can start to finesse it into more specific emotions. For example, within the category of happiness, you might distinguish between joy, contentment, pride or amusement. Within sadness, you might differentiate between disappointment, grief, loneliness or regret.

This process of finessing your emotions can be aided by expanding your emotional vocabulary. Just as an artist uses a variety of shades and tones, having a rich and nuanced emotional vocabulary allows you to describe your feelings with greater accuracy and specificity. It's the difference between knowing you're feeling good and understanding that you're feeling elated, grateful or serene.

On the Inside

Like me, you were probably taught that you have five senses: sight (visual), hearing (auditory), taste (gustatory), touch (tactile) and smell (olfactory). But you have an additional three: balance (vestibular), movement (proprioception) and internal (interoception). All of them are important, but when it comes to emotions and how you feel, interoception is the one that we need to understand.

Interoception is your ability to identify, understand and respond to internal bodily sensations. Interoceptive awareness refers to the conscious perception of sensations from inside the body, such as heartbeat, respiration, satiety (feeling full) and the autonomic sensations that are often associated with emotional reactions. When you feel thirsty or sense that you need to go to the toilet, that's down to your interoceptive awareness. Interoception is how you receive and perceive internal bodily signals, and how you're able to determine when you're thirsty, hungry, hot, cold, tired, alert, nauseous or even experiencing pain.

Some people have a greater degree of interoceptive awareness than others. As is the case with all the sensory systems, interoception can be impacted or impaired in those who are autistic, and those with poor interoceptive awareness may not be aware that they are cold, hungry or that their bladder is full and that they need to go to the toilet.

Interoception has a strong relationship with your SRS (see pages 1–2), because it's what enables your SRS to pick up on potential threats so well (although it's been suggested that if you are already experiencing significant stress then it can alter the intensity at which you experience internal interoceptive cues, as well as your perception and interpretation of them).

Several emotion theories emphasise the relevance of predicted bodily changes for the construction of one's own emotions. These theories are often grounded in the concept of embodied cognition, which posits that our thoughts, emotions and behaviours are deeply influenced by bodily sensations.

Experiencing emotion impacts your behaviour, but emotions are also a *consequence* of behaviour. The theory of emotion, proposed in 1884 by psychologists William James and Carl Lange, suggests that our emotional experiences are reactions to physiological changes in our bodies. For example, if you become aware that your body is trembling, you might interpret that as fear and say that you feel afraid. James, though, argued that it would be more accurate to say, 'I am afraid, because I have used my brain to assess that I am trembling and that this is a response to fear.'

I've seen this in action myself. In my previous work as a birth doula, I supported hundreds of women while they gave birth. After their baby was born, many of them experienced uncontrollable shaking and teeth chattering, like how you shiver when you feel cold. This, especially after the intensity of childbirth, usually freaked them out and I would witness a level of panic in their eyes and expression. However, as an experienced doula, I knew that this is a common bodily response to giving birth and can even be beneficial. As soon as I explained this to them, panic would transform into relief (and all the other emotions that hit post-birth), so even though the shaking continued, the knowledge that it's a normal and common response removed their fear and panic (though perhaps not the panic that they were now responsible for a tiny human being!).

The two-factor theory, also known as the Schachter-Singer theory, suggests that our emotions come from both our body's physiological reaction and how our mind interprets those reactions. Here's how it works: something happens, our body reacts and then we assess things cognitively. In other words, the physical sensation alone is not enough; to experience an emotion, we also need to identify the reason for this sensation.

Recent neuroscientific research supports these theories by showing an extensive overlap of brain regions involved during the perception of emotion intensity and the receiving, processing and interpretation of information from sensory receptors in the body. For instance, the insular cortex, a region involved in interoceptive awareness, is also implicated in the experience of emotions. The anterior cingulate cortex, another region associated with interoception, is also involved in processing emotional stimuli.

Research has also shown that improving interoceptive awareness can enhance the intensity of emotional experiences and improve emotional regulation. Poor interoceptive awareness is also associated with difficulties in regulating emotions, which makes a lot of sense, because emotions create bodily responses and lack of interoceptive awareness will make it more challenging to detect and work with them. However, don't go thinking that struggling to feel your emotions is solely about interoceptive ability – remember, very few of us have been taught to do this. This suggests that interventions aimed at improving interoceptive awareness, such as mindfulness-based therapies, could be beneficial for individuals with emotional disorders by addressing the following issues:

- Attention regulation: Mindfulness teaches individuals to focus their attention on the present moment. By practising this focus, you can learn to divert your attention away from ruminative or distressing thoughts, reducing their negative impact.
- Emotion regulation: By becoming more aware of your thoughts and feelings, you can recognise negative emotional patterns early on and use techniques to prevent them from escalating.
- Decreased reactivity: Mindfulness promotes a non-judgemental observation of thoughts and emotions. Over time, this can help reduce automatic, often negative, reactions to certain triggers or thoughts.
- Acceptance and non-judgement: Mindfulness encourages acceptance of one's feelings and thoughts without judgement. This perspective shift can decrease the intensity and duration of negative emotional episodes.
- Stress reduction: Mindfulness practices, especially meditation, have been shown to reduce the physiological and psychological markers of stress, leading to overall well-being.

Fostering awareness of bodily sensations is central to increasing interoception. I encourage my clients to take a moment to describe what they feel on a sensory level – they might describe a tightness in their throat, a warmth across their chest or a tension in their lower abdomen. This can be done while experiencing significant emotions as well as at random points in your day. I like to take note of what I'm feeling while waiting for the kettle to boil, when I'm sat in traffic or as I'm doing the dishes. There are plenty of opportunities to get curious about what you're feeling and experiencing, but the key is to pay attention without judgement. Other techniques that you can experiment with include:

- Guided visualisation exercises: These prompt you to imagine scenarios or experiences that can invoke strong bodily reactions, helping you to become more aware of your body's responses to emotions and thoughts.
- Mindful movement practices: Yoga, tai chi and walking meditations, for example, involve making intentional and slow body movements while paying attention to sensations and can enhance interoceptive awareness.
- Paying detailed attention to the experience of eating: The taste, texture, temperature and even the sounds of food can help improve interoceptive awareness by highlighting the sensations associated with hunger, fullness and taste.

Improving interoceptive awareness can help you to better understand your emotions as they manifest in the body, providing a tangible and often early signal of emotional distress. By catching and addressing these signals before they take hold, you can manage and regulate your emotions more effectively. However, as with most things in life, the pendulum can swing in the other direction and you can have heightened interoceptive awareness, which can be both advantageous and problematic, depending on the context and how it's managed.

Individuals with heightened interoception often have a keen understanding of their physical and emotional states, which can be beneficial in activities that require a high degree of self-awareness and understanding of the body, such as athletic endeavours. Those with enhanced interoceptive abilities might have a richer emotional experience that can be helpful in activities and professions that require deep empathy or emotional intelligence and expression.

However, someone who is constantly and acutely aware of their internal sensations might feel overwhelmed by the sheer volume and intensity of the information, and they may be labelled as hypochondriacs. Heightened awareness can also lead to exaggerated reactions to minor changes in your internal state; 'small' fluctuations in heart rate or discomforts that others might not notice or be able to overlook can become sources of anxiety, rumination and worry, making it hard to focus on the external world and tasks. Take it from someone who knows – while heightened interoceptive awareness can present challenges, with the right tools and understanding it's possible to harness its benefits.

Emotional Intensity

Emotions vary in intensity. What might start as a whisper of self-consciousness can quickly evolve into embarrassment, shame or even humiliation. Likewise, a gentle hum of satisfaction can bloom into contentment and happiness. The key to catching these emotional shifts early on is tuning into your interoceptive awareness.

Interoception is like your body's radio station, broadcasting the latest updates on your internal state. But here's the thing: if you're not used to tuning into this station, you might only pick up on the loudest signals. You might need an emotion to be blasting at an eight out of 10 before you notice it, or for it to be causing such a ruckus in your behaviour that it's impossible to ignore. But what if you could catch that broadcast when it's still a murmur, maybe a two or four out of 10? This is where honing your interoceptive awareness comes in. The insular cortex, a part of your brain that's like the radio receiver for your body's broadcasts, plays a crucial role in this process.

Practices like mindfulness can help you fine-tune this awareness, allowing you to pick up on these quieter broadcasts. This early detection system gives you the chance to recognise, process and interpret your emotional experiences before they reach full volume. It's like getting a heads-up that a song you don't like is about to play, giving you the chance to fully appreciate it, hear its message, change the station or adjust the volume.

This early detection system isn't about avoiding the 'bad' songs, it's about giving you more control over your emotional playlist. By catching these emotional shifts early, you have more opportunities to work with your emotions, deciding which ones you want to turn up; which ones you want to turn down; and which ones you want to listen to in full. Being responsive to your interoceptive cues can tip you off to the emergence of an emotion, giving you the space to recognise, process and interpret your experience, all of which gives you room to work out what you want to do about it.

When your emotional playlist is on mute

Alexithymia, a term coined by Dr Peter Sifneos in 1972, describes a unique emotional experience where an individual struggles to identify and articulate their emotions. This Greek term literally means having no words for emotions (a = lack, lexis = word, thymos = emotions). It isn't a diagnosis, but rather a way to describe someone's emotional experience. Alexithymia can manifest as an inability to recognise emotions, so someone might feel a surge of emotion, but can't pinpoint what they're feeling. It can also show up as a struggle to notice the subtle differences between various emotional states.

About 10 per cent of the population experience alexithymia to a high degree. It's associated with autism, ADHD and mental health conditions, including depression, eating disorders and schizophrenia. It's also seen in individuals who've had a stroke or experienced traumatic brain injury. In fact, researchers have identified two aspects of alexithymia: a cognitive dimension, which involves difficulties identifying, verbalising and analysing feelings, and an affective dimension, which includes challenges in reacting to, expressing and experiencing emotions.

Here's something else to consider: alexithymia isn't just about having no words for emotions; it's also about having fewer connections to emotions. Research has shown that individuals with high levels of alexithymia may have differences in the neural pathways involved in emotional processing, including reduced connectivity between regions involved in emotion generation and those involved in emotion regulation.

So, if you're someone who struggles to put your emotions into words, know that you're not alone. There are resources and strategies available to help you build your emotional vocabulary and connect more deeply with your emotional world *if* you want to and it feels useful to you – remember that recognising or naming emotions is just one way of understanding oneself and the world. The ability or inclination to do so is not inherently better or more evolved; everyone's emotional journey and capacity is valid and deserving of respect.

When your emotions are a technicolour symphony

Synaesthesia, in its most vibrant sense, is like a grand orchestra playing in your senses. It's a fascinating phenomenon where the stimulation of one sensory or cognitive pathway leads to automatic, involuntary experiences in a second sensory or cognitive pathway.

Imagine hearing a C-sharp on a piano, but not just hearing it – you see it too, as a burst of royal blue. Or perhaps the days of the week have their own distinct colours in your mind's eye – Monday is red, Tuesday is green and so on. That's synaesthesia.

Synaesthesia comes in many forms, with some of the most common types being grapheme-colour synaesthesia (where letters or numbers are perceived as inherently coloured), chromesthesia (where sounds, music or voices evoke the perception of colour), and lexical-gustatory synaesthesia (where certain words or sounds trigger taste sensations).

Now, imagine this in the context of emotions. Just as a C-sharp on a piano might trigger a burst of royal blue for a synesthete, an emotion might also evoke a sensory experience. This could be a colour, a taste or even a physical sensation. For instance, happiness might not just be a feeling, but a warm, golden glow spreading through your body. Anxiety might not just be an emotion, but a prickly, icy sensation creeping up your spine. This is emotional synaesthesia. It's not as widely studied as other forms, but it's a fascinating area of research and a valuable reminder that emotions aren't just abstract concepts, they're deeply intertwined with our sensory experiences. They're not just something we feel, but something we might also see, hear, taste or touch.

Research suggests that synaesthesia might be due to increased connectivity or communication between different areas of the brain, specifically those involved in processing sensory information. It's also thought to have a genetic component, as it tends to run in families. Synaesthesia is like a private concert of the senses, playing a symphony that's unique to each individual. It's a beautiful reminder that our emotional experiences are as diverse and complex as the symphony of senses that accompanies them.

The Beach Ball of Emotions

Picture a beach ball. It's colourful, it's bouncy, it's hard to ignore. Now, imagine that this beach ball symbolises all the emotions that you're feeling; the ones that don't feel great and the ones you'd rather not deal with. So, you head into the water and try to push the ball down under the water, but every time you try, it pops right back up. You try to press it down harder, but the more energy you exert, the more energy it has to pop back up, knocking you off balance.

But there's another way. Instead of trying to suppress the beach ball, picture yourself sitting quietly with it, gently holding it and getting to know it. It might feel strange at first, maybe even a bit uncomfortable, but by experiencing it and understanding it, you're able to locate the valve and release all the air.

This is what it means to truly experience your emotions – not to push them away or try to control them, but to sit with them, to understand them and, ultimately, to let them go. It's not always easy, but it's an essential part of emotional well-being. So next time you find yourself wrestling with a beach ball of emotions, remember: don't burst the bubble, embrace it. And if you're wondering how, don't worry. I got you covered...

Emotional Cartography

Embarking on the journey of processing emotions begins with a simple, yet profound step: mapping the landscape of your feelings. Start by noticing your physical experience of the emotion. Where do you feel it? Is it a tightness in your chest, a lump in your throat, a flutter in your stomach? Maybe it's a tension in your shoulders or a tingling in your hands. Are there areas that are being activated or lighting up or responding in some way? Is it more at the front of your body, your back or in the middle? Each emotion has its own unique physical signature and by tuning into these sensations, you can start to map the landscape of your feelings.

As you explore this emotional terrain, you might notice changes in your heart rate, breath and temperature. These are like the weather patterns of your emotional world, shifting and changing with each passing feeling. Now, as you notice where you feel the emotion, what do you notice about it? What qualities does it have? The brain likes to spin stories here and that's okay – that's just what brains do. But try to stick to the sensory experience of it. Think of yourself as an emotional explorer, curious and open to whatever you might discover. Here are some prompts to guide your journey:

- Does it feel empty or full?
- Does it shrink or expand?
- Is it small or big?

- Does it have a colour?
- Is it soft or hard or something else?
- Is it concentrated in a particular area?
- Does it spread out or do something else?
- Does it go inward, outward, up or down?
- If it moves, does it travel in a particular direction?
- Does it evolve or transform?

And finally, ask yourself: does this emotion bring a message with it? Is there something it wants to say or do? What's the urge or impulse that's there? How can you honour that? Remember, emotions are like messengers, each one carrying its own unique piece of information. By tuning into these messages, you can learn to navigate your emotional world with greater ease and understanding.

You've Got a Friend in Me

In our increasingly individualistic society, there's often a strong emphasis on self-reliance and independence. We're frequently told that strength lies in 'going it alone' and handling our problems by ourselves. This mindset, while sometimes beneficial, can also be harmful when it comes to processing our emotions. The truth is, we're not meant to navigate our emotional world in isolation. We are inherently social creatures and we thrive on connection.

Our emotions are deeply intertwined with our social interactions and relationships. This is why social support plays such a crucial role in processing emotions. Social support can come in many forms, from a comforting conversation with a close friend to professional help from a therapist or even the shared experience of a support group. These social connections provide a safe space for us to express and explore our emotions, and they can also offer valuable perspectives and advice.

One key aspect of social support in emotional processing is co-regulation, which is a process where individuals mutually influence each other's emotional states. It's a dynamic interplay that happens when we interact with others, especially those we are close to, including furry friends! Think about a time when you were feeling stressed or upset, and a calm and supportive friend was able to help you relax and feel better. That's co-regulation in action. Your friend's calm emotional state influenced your own, helping you to regulate your emotions more effectively.

Co-regulation is particularly important in early childhood development, but it doesn't stop there. Adults also benefit from co-regulating relationships. Having supportive people in our lives who can help us navigate our emotional landscape is invaluable. These relationships can provide a sense of comfort and stability, especially during challenging times.

The belief in individualism as superior can sometimes lead us to neglect these important social connections and support systems. But research has shown that social support and co-regulation can have a significant impact on mental health. Not to mention the lived experience of collectively experiencing a global pandemic that resulted in isolation for many.

People with strong social support networks are more resilient in the face of stress and adversity, and they are less likely to develop mental health disorders such as depression and anxiety. So, as you embark on your journey towards emotional proficiency, remember the importance of social support. Reach out to the people in your life and don't hesitate to seek professional help if you need or want it.

Chapter 7

Decisions

Every day we're faced with countless decisions, from the mundane – like what to have for breakfast – to the life-changing – like whether to take that job offer or move to a new city. Each decision we make shapes our lives in some way, big or small. But decision-making isn't just about choosing between option A or option B. It's also about how we handle the process of decision making and who we become as a result of making those changes. And let's be honest, sometimes that process can feel downright stressful. Ever felt like you're on the edge of a cliff and one wrong step could send you tumbling down? That's your stress response system kicking in, turning every decision into a high-stakes game. In this chapter, we're going to explore how stress affects our decision-making abilities and what we can do to navigate those high-pressure moments. We'll delve into the science behind it all and before you know it, you'll be a master of decision-making!

More is Less

Have you ever found yourself in a restaurant, staring at an extremely large menu with endless options and feeling utterly overwhelmed? Welcome to the paradox of choice. This concept, first used by psychologist Barry Schwartz, suggests that while we might think having plenty of options is a good thing, it can actually lead to decision paralysis.

So why does this happen? Well, when we're faced with too many choices, our brain goes into overdrive trying to evaluate every single option. It's like trying to juggle too many balls at once – eventually they all come crashing down. This can lead to feelings of overwhelm and anxiety, and in some cases we might avoid making a decision altogether.

And then there's the fear factor. When you're scared of making the wrong choice, the fear can paralyse you. It's like standing on the edge of a diving board, looking down at the water below and being too scared to jump, so you freeze. We worry about the consequences of our decisions and this fear can cause us to freeze, preventing us from making a choice at all.

Having too many options can simply be overwhelming. Our brains are not designed to handle a massive amount of information at once. When presented with too many choices, our cognitive load increases, making it harder for us to process information and make a decision, especially if we're already feeling stressed.

Stress

Stress can significantly affect how you make decisions. When your SRS is activated, you might feel a sense of urgency; a need to make a decision immediately or else face some kind of disaster that will be all your fault; or you could feel stuck and overwhelmed. It's easy to get swept up in this state and start blowing things out of proportion, making the situation seem more critical than it is, which only adds to your stress, creating a vicious cycle.

Sometimes this pressure will originate from an external source – you might receive an email from your team manager that states, 'This is really important, I need this NOW' and you could inadvertently take on their urgency. At other times, this will be water off a duck's back and what they say (and how they say it) will have little effect on you.

It's harder to think clearly when your SRS has jumped into 'We just need to get through this' survival mode. It pushes you into binary thinking, where there's a 'right' decision and a 'wrong' decision, and making the wrong choice feels like a life-or-death situation. This might sound dramatic, but it's how your SRS operates. As far as it's concerned, it's better to be extreme about things and survive than be nonchalant and die. But when you're operating in survival mode, you can't see all the options available and perfectionism comes in, because you're trying to get things right in order to stay safe.

However, this survival mode can limit your perspective. You might not be able to see all the options available to you and you might find yourself striving for perfection, trying to make the 'right' decision to stay safe. Remember, though, it's not about making the perfect decision, it's about making a decision that's good enough and allows you to move forward.

Don't Ask What I Want for Dinner

When you feel overwhelmed and want to run away from the responsibilities of life, the last thing you want is to be wandering the aisles of the supermarket, trying to figure out what to make for dinner. And don't get me started on being asked what I want for dinner, because when I'm feeling overwhelmed I just need the food to be put in front of me. In fact, when I'm feeling like this, I tell my family that I'm not available for questions. That can be easier said than done, because my kid is currently six years old (to be fair, not asking me questions can also prove challenging for my partner, who is 46, but that doesn't mean anything about him, because humans ask each other questions), so I let my son know that I'm finding questions hard.

When the demands of life feel like they're more than you have capacity for, you might experience a temporary sense of hopelessness and either want things to go away (I call this going into ostrich mode) or want other people to decide for you. It's essentially a form of giving up and there's nothing wrong with that. It may not be what you want to happen, but it could be what you need. They probably won't make the decision that you would if you were feeling regulated and capable, but there are times when what's best in that moment is to take it off your plate, giving yourself time out while your body and brain come back online again. This is when taking more time *is* beneficial.

Your ability to make decisions is closely tied to the state of your nervous system. When your nervous system is regulated and you feel safe, you're able to make decisions effectively and efficiently. You can see the broader picture and determine the real issue. It's an expansive way of looking at things that also enables you to think creatively and come up with unique solutions. Your choices will be goal-oriented.

However, while making decisions when you're in a stress response state isn't wrong, your choice will be about getting through things rather than being goal-oriented. In a state of overwhelm you could find yourself feeling stuck or unable to make decisions. Rather than berating yourself for struggling to make what would ordinarily be a simple decision, like what to have for dinner, see it as a protective response designed to help you conserve energy and survive in the face of perceived threats. When you're in a state of hypoarousal (see pages 46–8), it can take some time for our body to come back online and for us to regain our capacity for decision-making. Knowing that there is a physiological reason for this helps you to accept that there are times when you just can't make a decision and to give yourself time to come around.

When you're feeling this way, going along with what others decide can be a form of self-protection. It can feel safer and less energy-consuming to let others make decisions for you, especially if you're struggling to process information or weigh up options. This is particularly true if the decisions are about non-threatening or everyday matters, like what to have for dinner.

Fawning Over Decisions

The fawn response, also known as please-and-appease (see pages 89–90) is characterised by people-pleasing behaviour, where the individual attempts to avoid conflict, criticism or abandonment by going out of their way to please others, often at the expense of their own needs or well-being. In terms of decision-making, individuals who tend to exhibit the fawn response may struggle to make decisions that prioritise their own needs and desires. They may be overly concerned with the opinions or desires of others, leading to indecisiveness or decisions that they later regret. Responses that are suggestive of the fawn response include:

- I just don't mind.
- Either way – you decide.
- Whatever you want is fine with me.
- But what would you like to do?
- Oh no, you decide.
- Whatever you want is fine.

These can also be genuine responses in the sense that there will be times when you truly don't mind or don't have a preference. There are things that I just don't have a strong opinion about or situations where either option is acceptable. When my partner presents them to me and asks what do I want to do, I'm genuinely good with whatever he wants to do, but I'm not people-pleasing when I'm doing that, I'm being very genuine in my not being fussed. If it's something that he cares about then it makes much more sense to be guided by him. And trust me, there are plenty of things that I have very strong preferences about.

While there are endless benefits to empathy and cooperation in personal and professional relationships, people-pleasing is different to considering the needs and preferences of others. They might look the same on the outside, but internally they differ. The key is to strike a balance, ensuring that your own needs and desires are also being met.

Fifty Shades of Grey

Cognitive distortions – irrational thought patterns that can skew your perception of reality – have a significant impact on decision-making. Let's explore how (for a more complete list of cognitive distortions, see pages 26–7).

All-or-nothing thinking

This is when we see things in black and white, with no middle ground. In the context of decision-making, this can lead us to believe that there's a 'right' decision and a 'wrong' decision, with no room for nuance, causing stress and making it harder to make a decision. When my client Lauren was offered a job in another city, she got stuck in an all-or-nothing mindset.

She told me, *'If I take this job and move, it means I'm completely turning my back on my friends and family here. But if I stay, it means I'm passing up on every professional opportunity out there.'* This rigid way of thinking prevented her from considering more nuanced possibilities, like the idea that she could take the job and still maintain strong ties with her current community, or that there might be other, equally good job opportunities in the future which wouldn't require relocation. Lauren framed her decision as a stark choice between personal life and professional growth, rather than exploring a balanced approach.

Overgeneralisation

This is when we take one event or piece of evidence and generalise it to an overall pattern. For example, if we made a bad decision in the past, we might think we're bad at making decisions in general. This can undermine our confidence and make it harder to make decisions in the future. For example, after choosing a restaurant that served disappointing food and had terrible service, you jump to, 'I *always* pick the wrong places. Someone else should make these decisions. They'd *never* make a mistake like this.'

Catastrophising

This is when we imagine the worst possible outcome. In decision-making, this can lead us to inflate the potential negative consequences of a decision, causing unnecessary stress and fear, which then makes it harder to make a decision that's goal-focused. Instead, you'll make a threat-focused decision.

Let's say you're considering applying for a promotion at work. Instead of focusing on the potential benefits or growth, you begin to imagine all the things that could go wrong. You start to think, 'If I apply and don't get it, everyone will see me as incompetent. My colleagues will lose respect for me and laugh at me. Maybe my manager will think I'm not even fit for my current role and will start considering letting me go. I might end up jobless.' This line of thinking causes so much distress that you decide not to apply at all, even though you're well-qualified for the promotion. The decision becomes more about avoiding the imagined worst-case scenario than about achieving a potential career milestone.

Discounting the positive

This is when we ignore or downplay positive information. If we're deciding whether to take on a new challenge, for example, we might discount our past successes and focus only on the potential for failure. When you successfully navigate nine out of 10 challenges in planning an event, but dwell on one mistake or oversight, you think it ruined everything, yet nobody else is bothered by it. In fact, they probably didn't even notice it.

Mind-reading

This one's a biggie. It's when we assume that we know what others are thinking. In decision-making, this can lead us to make decisions based on what we think others want or expect, rather than what's best for us.

Mind-reading can be particularly prevalent in those socialised as female, thanks to societal norms and expectations. From a young age, girls are often socialised to be attuned to the needs and feelings of others, sometimes at the expense of their own. This can lead to a tendency to try and anticipate what others are thinking or expecting, and to adjust our behaviour accordingly. It's like we're trying to be mind-readers and people-pleasers all at once.

This makes decision-making especially tricky. If you're constantly trying to guess what others want or expect from us, you'll lose sight of what you truly want or need. Making decisions based on your assumptions about others' expectations, rather than your own desires and values, leads to feelings of resentment, dissatisfaction and a loss of authenticity. And most of the time, we have no clue if our assumptions are even correct.

The key to overcoming this cognitive distortion is to recognise when you're doing it and to remind yourself that you can't read minds. If knowing what others think and feel is important to you, then try asking them.

Emotion Commotion

Emotions play a significant role in decision-making. They can influence our choices, act as shields and even paralyse us with fear or uncertainty. But here's the thing: our emotions aren't something to be feared or avoided. They're a natural part of being human and they can provide valuable insights if we're willing to listen.

Accepting and managing our emotions is a crucial part of decision-making. When we try to ignore or suppress our emotions, they can end up controlling us. But when we acknowledge and accept our emotions, we can make more conscious, intentional decisions.

This doesn't mean we should let our emotions dictate our decisions. Rather, it means recognising our emotions, understanding how they're influencing us and then making a decision that aligns with our values and goals.

Emotional Shields

Experiencing confusion or uncertainty when faced with a decision is central to the human experience. These emotions will feel very real to you and they are, but be honest with yourself: are you confused or are you scared of how others will react to your decision? Are you uncertain about what to do or is uncertainty protecting you from doubting yourself?

Confusion and uncertainty can act as shields, protecting us from confronting potentially uncomfortable emotions. For instance, if a decision might lead to a confrontation, we might feel confused or uncertain in order to avoid feeling fear or anxiety. However, these shields can also hinder our decision-making process, as they prevent us from fully understanding our emotional responses to different choices.

My client Katie realised that being undecided about having kids was an attempt to shield herself from other emotions. She says, *I've been "undecided" for years, but that's really hiding my fears of being left alone with a child as my partner doesn't really want kids or having kids and feeling like I've made a mistake. Most decisions you can change your mind on, but having kids and regretting it is not one of them! I'd cope if it came to that, but I'm sat in indecision to avoid my fears.'*

Abbie had a similar journey. She was offered an incredible job opportunity abroad. On the surface she told herself and everyone around her that she was 'confused' about whether to take the job. *'I love my life here,'* she'd say, *'so I'm uncertain if moving is the right choice.'* But after some soul-searching and coaching, Abbie realised her confusion was a smokescreen for her real feelings. She shared, *'I'm not confused about the job. I know it's a golden opportunity. What I'm terrified of is the loneliness I might feel being so far from family and my tight-knit circle of friends. I've never been good at making new friends. My "uncertainty" was really me avoiding confronting that deep-seated fear of isolation.'*

Abbie's story underscores how our minds can cleverly disguise raw, vulnerable feelings with the more socially acceptable sentiments of confusion or uncertainty. Sometimes, it's about peeling back the layers and being brutally honest to unearth what's really holding us back.

Fear of Success and Fear of Failure

Interestingly, both the fear of success and the fear of failure can impact our decision-making. Fear of success might seem counterintuitive, but it's a real phenomenon and one I see a lot among my clients. Some people might fear success because they worry about the increased responsibilities, expectations or changes that could come with it. On the other hand, fear of failure can lead people to avoid taking risks or making decisions that could potentially lead to failure, even if those decisions could also lead to significant rewards.

Riding the Hormonal Rollercoaster

The monthly hormonal dance of the menstrual cycle has a significant impact on your decision-making abilities. It's like having a hormonal board of directors in your brain, each member with a different perspective on how to handle the situation.

Oestrogen: the optimist

When oestrogen levels are high, it's like having a cheerleader in your brain. 'It'll be fantastic! Everything will work out brilliantly! The world is wonderful!' Higher levels of oestrogen are linked to higher levels of dopamine, which impacts learning and reward. This can lead to a more optimistic outlook and the confidence and willingness to take on challenges.

Testosterone: the risk-taker

Testosterone is the board member that's all about taking risks and seizing the moment. 'Take a risk! Go for it! It's now or never!' This hormone can make you more competitive and willing to take risks.

Progesterone: the prudent

Progesterone is the cautious member of the board. When progesterone levels rise, it's like having a voice in your head saying, 'What the hell were you thinking when you decided to do that? That's the worst idea ever. You should just stay inside where it's safe and stick your head in the sand and wait it out. Let someone else decide for you.' This hormone can make you more cautious and risk-averse, especially if your inner critic has a lot to say when you're premenstrual.

While you can make a decision at any point in your cycle, it's useful to consider how your hormones could be influencing your choice. The best way to do this is by getting to know your experience of your cycle by tracking it. You can read all about this in my book, *Period Power*, and you can use the free cycle-tracking guide available through my website (www.maisiehill.com/chartmycycle). Each part of the cycle offers a different perspective, but rather than using this to hold you back from making decisions, use it to inform those decisions.

Under Pressure

What implicit and explicit messages about making decisions did you absorb in your childhood and as you grew up?

- You should take your time
- It's hard and complicated
- There's a right decision and a wrong one
- You must consider other people's feelings
- You must consider other people's needs
- Once a decision's been made, there's no going back
- It's better to go with the safe option
- Everyone must be happy with your decision
- Listen to the people in positions of authority
- Everything needs to be weighed up very carefully
- You need to do a lot of research
- Impulsivity is not a good thing
- Always have a plan B
- It's important to really think it through.

No wonder so many of us struggle to make decisions and feel under pressure to make the right one!

Our caregivers play a significant role in shaping our decision-making abilities, so what was your experience of making decisions as you grew up: Were you given opportunities to make them or did other people make them for you? Did you get to experience the consequences of your decisions or did your caregivers save or rob you of those opportunities? Was failure unacceptable and were you shamed for making the 'wrong' choice? Or did you grow up in an environment where failing was accepted and encouraged? Was research and the gathering of information prioritised over your gut sense of what decision to make? These early experiences can have a lasting impact on how we approach decision-making as adults and understanding how they've influenced you provides opportunities to unwind unhelpful beliefs and behaviours, and forge new ones.

Like many of my clients, you may have made decisions for yourself, only to be overruled by your parents. You might have wanted to keep your parents happy (or to avoid their wrath) or witnessed a hierarchy of who gets the final say in the household that meant you and other members of the household always deferred to them.

Don't Believe Everything You Think

When it comes to decisions, there are some thoughts that I see in my clients (and myself) time and time again that will always stand in the way and it gives me great pleasure to dismantle these absolute whoppers for you.

What if I make the wrong decision?

What if you do? Really answer that question. It's not a problem that this question appears in your head, but not answering it will cause issues. First of all, if it goes unanswered then it'll remain as a vague threat, but if you give a specific answer then you'll have something you can work with.

The bigger point here is that there is a presumption that there *is* a right decision, but actually there's no such thing as a right decision. And yes, of course there are times where there is a right or wrong decision – if you're performing surgery on someone, for example. But I'm sure the surgeons among you would tell me that there's nuance in the operating theatre, too.

The idea of a right or perfect choice is an illusion. There are usually multiple good options and the 'best' choice can depend on a variety of factors, many of which are unpredictable or out of our control, so while it's natural to want to make the best possible decision, it's important to remember that perfection is not always attainable or even necessary. Sometimes, 'good enough' is more than enough.

Instead of there being a right and a wrong decision, try reframing it as a decision that you make right or that you make wrong. You can also just decide that you've made the right decision – that's just a thought and it's completely in your control, which means that you can't get it wrong. If there's no right decision, then you can't get it wrong.

There's no going back – this decision is permanent

There are times when that's true, but often it isn't. You can change your mind; you can do things differently. When I catch myself doing that and thinking, 'Oh, this is a forever decision,' I've trained my brain to go to, 'No it's not, that's just a thought.' And instead, I think about how I can approach things with an air of experimentation instead. If I'm just experimenting and trying something out, so that I can see what I think about it, then that frees me up to think creatively about decisions.

I'm going to upset/offend/disappoint others

Yes, people will absolutely feel disappointed and upset with your decision. I know it's not what you want to hear, but it's true. So what? Most of the time, this is just our brains being dramatic with stuff, and trying to keep us safe and protect us. Great job, brain, but I like to use the 'and then what?' technique to take myself to the place of, well what if these things do happen? To use this technique, simply ask yourself 'and then what?' and for each answer that you come up with, ask 'and then what?' again. By doing this, you'll delve deeper into your fears and understand the root of your apprehension. Let's say that some people will be upset, offended or disappointed. And then what? They might shake their head, make a face, express their opinion verbally or send you a text. And then what? You'll have your thoughts and feelings about their response. And for the most part, that's probably about it.

And what if someone is upset, angry or disappointed? It's okay for people to feel upset and disappointed, and it's not only not your job to keep everyone happy, it's also not possible. This might be big news to you, but people also care far less than you think they do. They're too busy thinking about their own stuff to give two hoots about yours. Most of my clients are pleasantly surprised by the results of their hard conversations and they usually provide good evidence they're worth having and rarely as bad as you anticipate.

This is a once-in-a-lifetime opportunity

When you think this way, you're not seeing yourself as someone who creates their own opportunities. If you believe you must make this decision now, because you're not going to get a chance like it again, you're viewing life as something that happens to you. If you tell yourself these things are dependent on other people, fate, the universe or God, you're wrong. They're not. You will have plenty of opportunities and there are always more chances, especially if you see yourself as someone who creates them.

This is a BIG decision

According to whom? Who said it's a big decision? How do we know it's a big decision? How do we measure it? This is just a thought. It isn't factual and telling yourself that it's a big decision is unhelpful. I've yet to experience coaching someone who was helped by thinking about a decision as a big decision. Usually, it results in them feeling pressure, overwhelm and stress, so they end up in a stress response and they either want to run away and hide from it, or freeze and don't take any action at all. And while this is going on, it's deepening their belief that they can't make decisions, resulting in a situation where they're watching life pass them by.

While I highly recommend removing 'It's a big decision' from your vocabulary, it is helpful to explore why a decision feels big. You don't have to judge yourself and its size may be very logical and real for you. However, when my clients get rid of the idea that something is a big decision, they often realise that they do know what they want to do, but the thought that it was big was preventing them from engaging with their truth. My client Jo had been in a relationship for seven years and was trying to decide whether to break up or continue to work on things. She was struggling to decide and when I asked her why, she told me that it was a huge decision (a statement that she'd repeatedly told herself and her friends), so I simply asked her, 'What if it's not – even if it feels like it is?' When Jo set that notion that it was a big decision aside, she realised that she knew exactly what she wanted to do and ended the relationship.

I need more information

I suspect there's going to be quite a few of you who feel more comfortable in the research phase of a decision. And there are times when gathering information is useful, but those times are far fewer than you think. Researching is the comfortable part of making a decision, because you're not actually making the decision, taking action, or living with the consequences of the decision. If this sounds familiar, then be honest with yourself about what's going on. Again, you don't have to judge or criticise yourself for it, but it's helpful to be clear about how your brain is trying to get out of making the decision.

I need more time

For what? I'm serious. What will more time give you? Taking time to regulate your nervous system and address unhelpful thoughts is one thing, but even those helpful techniques can be used as an avoidance strategy. In most cases, delaying making a decision is going to take up mental real estate. When someone tells me they need more time to make a decision, 99 per cent of the time they have decided already, but it's uncomfortable for them to own that decision, so they put some time in front of them as a way to avoid taking action on what they have already decided on.

I need to sleep on it

Okay, I'll give you this one. Sometimes sleeping on it is useful. If you're experiencing fatigue or significant stress, then you can struggle to see things clearly, in which case sleeping on it can be a helpful strategy.

If I'm wrong, I'll waste time/energy/money/resources

We've already concluded that there's no such thing as a wrong decision, but, just for fun, let's go along with your brain: You made a decision and took action that led to you finding stuff out that you wouldn't have known had you not moved forward with things, and that now means that you can take a different course of action. And the more you do this, the quicker you will get to your desired result. How is that a waste? It sounds highly productive to me, but it does require you to increase your capacity for failure (I've got you covered on that front). And it may also mean that you do things in a leaner way, so that fewer resources are used along the way, and that will involve you dropping any perfectionist tendencies that you have (I've got you covered there, too).

I'll get told off

This one is a huge unnoticed thought that many of my clients have running very subtly in the background of their lives. And although your rational brain can recognise you probably won't – or if you are that you'll be able to handle it in an appropriate way – your nervous system could very well be on red alert.

Pros and Cons

In case you were wondering, a pros and cons list is *not* an effective way to make a decision. While there are times when it's helpful to understand the lie of the land and try to get a sense of the impact of a decision, the problem is that for every pro you'll find a con, and all that happens is the list gets longer.

The classic pros and cons list is a tool many of us turn to when faced with a tough decision. But is it helpful? It overemphasises logic which, although important, can come at the expense of the insights from emotions and intuition that logic can't capture. That can then lead to paralysis by analysis, where we get so caught up in analysing each option that we end up feeling overwhelmed and unable to make a decision. More information doesn't necessarily make it easier to decide.

Not all pros and cons are created equal, but when placed side by side they can end up being treated as if they were. This can lead us to overvalue minor factors and undervalue major ones. It can also cause us to lose track of the bigger picture. Instead, we focus too narrowly on the specifics of each option and in doing so fail to see other, potentially better, options.

However, the biggest issue that I see with lists of pros and cons is that they reinforce indecision, adding more and more items to each side of the list, without getting any closer to making a decision. What's really going on here is that you're using writing a list to delay or get out of making a decision. If, when you write out your pros and cons, the thoughts that are running in the background are 'I don't know what to do,' or 'I'm worried I'll make the wrong choice,' or 'It's so hard to make a decision,' then it's highly unlikely that you'll make one. Instead, you'll just have a long list of things that prevent you from making a decision and taking action.

It's also important to consider the nervous system state that you're in when that decision is presented to you, because if you are already dysregulated and in fight or flight or freeze, then that will dictate how you respond to a decision. It will be very different if you're feeling quite regulated and someone asks you to make a decision or, equally, if it's the end of a challenging day when you've been in a stress response and just want to switch off.

Face the Truth

I can't tell you the number of times where I've been coaching a client who's struggling to make a decision, but as we explore what's going on it becomes clear that they made a decision quickly, but it felt uncomfortable, so instead of sticking with the discomfort, understanding it and moving through it, they backtrack. We've all been there. You've made a decision, but then you start to second-guess yourself and come up with reasons why maybe it isn't the right choice, and you try to talk yourself out of it. This is where honesty comes into play. Being honest with yourself means acknowledging what you truly want or believe, even if it's uncomfortable or scary. It means facing your fears, your doubts and your insecurities, and standing by your decision despite them.

The next time you find yourself trying to talk yourself out of a decision, take a moment to reflect. Ask yourself: 'Have I already made a decision? Or am I just trying to talk myself out of it?' If the answer is yes, then it's time to embrace your decision and move forward.

Double Trouble: Cognitive Dissonance

Cognitive dissonance is a theory that was proposed by Leon Festinger in 1957. It refers to the mental discomfort that a person feels when they hold two or more contradictory beliefs, values or attitudes, especially in a situation where they have made a decision that conflicts with their previous beliefs, values or identity.

In the context of decision-making, cognitive dissonance can occur when a person has made a choice, but then experiences doubt or regret about it, leading them to try and rationalise their decision or talk themselves out of it. This can be due to fear of making the wrong decision, fear of the potential consequences or a desire to avoid discomfort or change.

For instance, imagine you've always cherished the closeness of family, but an enticing job opportunity abroad presents itself. While the allure of a new adventure might initially captivate you, the acceptance of such a role could stir internal conflict, especially with thoughts of leaving behind ageing parents and a familiar community. In a more everyday context, consider a day where despite a lengthy to-do list, you're drawn into binge-watching your favourite series. To prevent your partner from discovering this diversion, you might go to lengths to give the impression of a day filled with productivity.

Step by Step

Life is a lot like a staircase. Each decision we make is a step that takes us higher, closer to our goals. When you're faced with a decision, it's easy to get overwhelmed by all the potential outcomes and consequences, and you might want to jump ahead to the tenth step, trying to predict what might happen down the line. But here's the thing: you can't leap up the entire staircase in one go. It's not only impossible, it's also exhausting and stressful, and you must take it one step at a time. My client Marie experienced this during a year in which many parts of her life began to change.

Client Story

Marie had moved home, was grieving the death of a friend and had managed to keep her job in the face of company-wide redundancies, but was experiencing burnout due to the increased workload and significant pressure around whether she'd keep her job or not. On top of that, she and her partner were discussing whether they would try to conceive. As Marie considered what the next few years of her life might be, she found it impossible to come up with a plan: Should she stay in her current role or transfer to another team? Or get a job elsewhere or maybe be self-employed? What if she was pregnant, wouldn't it be better to be employed and receive the company benefits and maternity pay? But then again, maybe being self-employed would be better, because she'd be able to manage her own schedule. What if she wasn't pregnant though? What about the PhD she was longing to do? Maybe now was the perfect time to do it, but what if she didn't get any funding and needed to pay for it? Then it would be better to have her current salary. But wouldn't being employed full-time make it harder for her to do her PhD?

Marie's scenario epitomises how, when faced with a flurry of life changes and decisions, we can easily find ourselves tangled in a web of endless 'what if' scenarios, trying to anticipate every potential outcome. Mapping out various scenarios like this is your brain's attempt to protect and prepare you, but this forward-projecting can become paralysing, leading to decision fatigue and inertia.

As I coached Marie, she realised that the most important decision wasn't any of the things that were on her list of things to decide. Her most important decision was to prioritise her health and focus on recovering from burnout. The past few months had taken a huge toll on her and she recognised that how she was feeling was not only getting in the way of being able to make decisions, but that it would limit her ability to actually carry out any plan that she came up with.

Marie spoke to her GP, who promptly signed her off work for three months. During this time she rested, recovered and, as her resilience returned, it became obvious to her what her next, best step was, and she was able to approach life with a sense of playfulness – a far cry from the pressure she'd been experiencing for so long. Marie discovered that rather than trying to find certainty where there is none to be found and having a perfect plan, what's most important is to take care of the first step, and to have the resilience and capacity to navigate whatever comes your way.

Focusing on the decision that's right in front of you is often the best step. Don't worry about the rest of the staircase for now. Just take that one step. Make that one decision. Be fully present in it. Once you've taken that step, then you can think about the next one. And then the next one. And so on. By taking it one step at a time, you'll find that the staircase isn't as daunting as it first seemed. Remember, you don't have to have it all figured out right now. You don't have to know exactly how everything will turn out. All you have to do is take the next step. This aligns with the concept of 'affective forecasting' proposed by psychologists Timothy Wilson and Daniel Gilbert, which suggests that we're often inaccurate in predicting our future emotional state.

So, the next time you're faced with a decision, don't let your brain leap ahead to the tenth step. Just focus on the decision that's in front of you. Take it one step at a time. You'll be amazed at how far you can climb.

Closing Tabs

Imagine your mind is a laptop and each decision you need to make is an open tab in your browser. Some tabs are more demanding than others – they are playing videos or running complex scripts – while others are just static pages. But no matter how simple, each open tab is using up some of your laptop's resources – its processing power, its memory and, most importantly, its battery life.

Now, think about how your laptop performs when you have too many tabs open. It slows down, right? It might even freeze or crash. And the battery drains faster than usual. That's exactly what happens to us when we're carrying around a load of unmade decisions. They're like those open tabs, quietly draining our mental energy and reducing our performance.

So, what's the solution? Just as you would close unnecessary tabs on your laptop to save battery, you need to deal with your decision baggage. Here's a simple strategy that I recommend for when you have a backlog of decisions that's taking up mental real estate: Set aside a dedicated period (say, 20 minutes) to power through those decisions. Make a list of all the decisions you're lugging around and tackle each one, one at a time.

During this time, your sole focus should be on making decisions. Don't worry about implementing them just yet. That's a task for future you. Right now, your job is to decide, but before you dive in, make sure you're setting yourself up for success by avoiding being hungry or feeling rushed. If you're hungry, your brain might be more focused on finding food than making decisions and feeling hungry has been known to have a deleterious influence on the ability to make decisions. And if you're feeling rushed, you might not give each decision the consideration it deserves. So, grab a snack, clear your schedule and then get down to business.

By the end of your decision-making session, you'll likely feel a sense of relief, similar to the satisfaction of closing all those extra tabs on your laptop. You've freed up mental resources and can now operate more efficiently. And who knows, with all that extra mental energy, you might just find that you're able to tackle bigger and more complex tasks with ease. Decision-making, like any other skill, takes practice. The more you do it, the better you'll get. Close those tabs, clear your decision baggage and see how much more smoothly your mental laptop runs.

Combat Decision Fatigue

Decision fatigue refers to the deteriorating quality of decisions made by an individual after a long session of decision-making. It's a psychological phenomenon in which making too many decisions can lead to mental exhaustion and reduced decision-making ability. This can result in either decision avoidance (where people postpone decisions or choose the default option) or impulsive decision-making (where people make hasty choices).

The concept was popularised by social psychologist Roy F. Baumeister and is based on the Freudian hypothesis of ego depletion or the loss of self-control after extended periods of exertion. It's a significant factor in cognitive overload, affecting productivity, mental well-being and even physical health. Understanding and managing decision fatigue can help you to make better choices, and maintain mental clarity, and I recommend that you explore whether it's making decisions that feels exhausting, or if it's the lack of making decisions and the associated pile-up of things that need to be decided that is weighing on you. Here are some strategies for reducing decision fatigue:

- Limit your choices: Having too many options can lead to decision paralysis, so try to limit your choices to a manageable number. This can be applied to anything from your wardrobe to your meal planning. My life got a lot easier when I started buying clothes from the same brands, because everything goes together.
- Prioritise your decisions: Not all decisions are created equal so prioritise the more important ones and spend less time on the low-stakes ones.
- Create rhythms and routines: Automating some of your daily decisions frees up mental energy. For example, having a set morning routine can eliminate the need to decide what to do when you first get up.
- Rest and recharge: Decision fatigue can be exacerbated by physical fatigue. Make sure you're getting enough sleep, eating well and taking breaks when needed.
- Accept imperfection: No decision is perfect and accepting this can take some of the pressure off and make decision-making less stressful.
- Delegate decisions: If possible, pass on some decisions to others. This can be particularly helpful in a work context, but I know plenty of households and romantic relationships that have benefited from it.

Lightening the Load

Delegating decisions is a powerful tool to help alleviate the mental and emotional burden of decision-making. Especially for women, who shoulder the double-burden of unpaid and paid labour in the home and in the professional environment. The disproportionate amount of responsibility adds up, as does the number of decisions we're required to make within the various roles we undertake: friend, daughter, sister, aunt, employee, manager, caregiver, cleaner, mother, organiser, calendar-keeper, gift-giver, tea-maker, reader of minds, and part-time therapist to all and sundry.

Now think about how many requests and individual decisions need to be made within each of those. No wonder so many women are exhausted, fed up and angry. My personal opinion is that the best decision one can make in circumstances like these is to decide that you are no longer available for all the above, at least not to the extent that you have been. Here are some examples from my clients of delegation in action:

- Work projects: Cynthia, a manager at a marketing firm, often felt overwhelmed with her responsibilities and her professional life was extremely demanding. She began to delegate specific tasks to her team members, trusting in their skills. Cynthia got team members to lead certain client meetings or to take charge of a segment of a project. This not only reduced her workload, but also empowered her team, leading to a more collaborative and efficient work environment.
- Social commitments: Sophia loves to prioritise her friendships, but ended up being the one constantly coordinating group gatherings, outings and trips with friends. While she loved being so connected to her social circle, the planning became a bit much. Sophia decided to suggest a rotation system. Every month, a different friend now takes charge of organising the group's main meetup. This not only reduced her planning burden, but also introduced the group to new experiences they might not have tried under her sole direction.
- Cleaning: Priyanka was a freelancer who struggled with managing her work-life balance. She was busy working from home during the day, but kept being distracted by the dishes and dust that had accumulated. At first, she was hesitant to add what she viewed as an unnecessary expense to her outgoings, but once I asked her what she could do with that time and how much money she could create with it, she decided to hire a cleaning service for deep cleaning sessions once a month, giving her a break and ensuring her home was thoroughly cleaned.
- Leveraging technology: Ella worked full-time and, although she wanted to eat homemade meals, by the time she reached the supermarket in

the evening, she was unable to decide what to make and found herself staring at the broccoli and asparagus. To simplify matters, she started using free meal-planning apps that generated weekly menus based on what she had in her pantry. This not only saved her time, but also reduced food waste.

- Household chores: After years of bearing the brunt of household decisions, Rina sat down with her partner and kids and told them she was no longer available to do this. She was clear and explicit about what she would be doing and stated that the rest was up to them.

Delegating decisions doesn't mean abdicating responsibility. It involves assessing all areas of your life, recognising where the burdens lie and finding practical ways to distribute that load, especially on individuals who might be juggling too much. Remember, it's not just about distributing tasks, but also about sharing the mental and emotional responsibility that comes with decision-making. For those used to carrying the weight, delegation can offer a refreshing and often necessary break.

A New Frame of Mind

Instead of viewing a decision as a life-or-death situation, try to see it as just one decision among many that you'll make in your life. This can help take some of the pressure off and make the decision feel less monumental. Remember, it's okay to make mistakes. In fact, every decision you make, however it turns out, is an opportunity to learn and grow.

Another helpful reframe is to shift your thinking from 'I have to decide' to 'I get to choose.' This subtle shift can make a big difference in how you approach decision-making. Instead of seeing it as a burden, you're acknowledging it as an opportunity and recognising that you have the power to shape your own life through the decisions you make.

This reframing technique is backed by research in cognitive psychology, which shows that how we frame or interpret situations can significantly impact our emotional and behavioural responses. So, the next time you're faced with a tough decision, try to reframe the situation. You might be surprised at how much it can help, just as my client Lara was.

She had been offered a new job, but kept changing her mind about whether to accept it or not, because, as she put it, 'There's so much to the decision –

time with my daughter, the commute to London, wages, career progression, as well as the issues in the company that I currently work for.' Rather than focusing on what decision to make, I encouraged Lara to look at how she was making the decision and she realised that her predominant thought was, 'I don't know what to do' – no wonder she was going around in circles and changing her mind all the time. Lara decided to feel excited about having options and to change her internal narrative to 'I know what to do.' This, in turn, made her feel focused on her long-term goals and her values, and she realised that, lo and behold, she did know what to do. Instead of accepting the job offer, she decided to apply for an internal role at her current company that excited her instead.

Embrace Uncertainty

Uncertainty is a natural part of decision-making. After all, we can't predict the future. We can't know for sure how things will turn out. We can gather information, weigh our options and make the best decision we can with the information we have. However, at the end of the day, there's always going to be some level of uncertainty.

Now, you might be thinking, 'Uncertainty sounds stressful, Maisie. Why would I want to embrace it?' Well, while uncertainty can be uncomfortable, it also has its benefits. Embracing uncertainty can free us from the pressure of having to make the 'perfect' decision. It can open us up to new possibilities and allow us to be more flexible and adaptable.

Research has shown that our brains are wired to seek certainty and avoid uncertainty. A study by University College London found that uncertainty can cause more stress than knowing something bad will definitely happen. This is because uncertainty triggers our fight-or-flight response, causing us to feel threatened. So, how can we manage uncertainty and make decisions despite it? Here are a few strategies:

- Practice acceptance: Accept that uncertainty is a part of life and a part of decision-making. You don't have to like it, but accepting it can reduce the stress and anxiety it causes. Get comfortable with not knowing.
- Take small steps: If uncertainty is making it hard for you to make a decision, try breaking it down into smaller decisions. This can make the decision-making process feel less overwhelming.

- Write about it: Get all your thoughts and feelings down on paper, so that you can see what's really going on. The key here is not to edit or censor yourself and to have self-compassion for what comes up.
- Reframe uncertainty: Instead of seeing uncertainty as a threat, try to see it as an opportunity. Uncertainty means that there are multiple possible outcomes, some of which could be better than you imagine. Get curious and have fun exploring what might happen.

Life is full of uncertainties and as much as you might want a crystal ball or clear signpost, the reality is that it's more like trying to navigate the world with a map that's constantly changing. Decision-making is inherently uncertain, but here's the thing: uncertainty isn't necessarily a bad thing. In fact, it can be a powerful ally in decision-making if we learn to embrace it rather than avoid it. Uncertainty keeps us open to new possibilities and allows us to approach decisions with a sense of curiosity and exploration, rather than fear and dread. It encourages us to question our assumptions, consider different perspectives and be flexible in our thinking, all of which are valuable tools when it comes to making decisions. Research has shown that people who are comfortable with uncertainty are less likely to fall into cognitive biases, such as overconfidence or confirmation bias, and are more likely to be creative and innovative, as they're not constrained by a rigid need for certainty.

A cognitive bias is when our brains play a little trick on us, drawing us away from the straight path of logic. Think of it as a mental shortcut or a little hiccup in our thinking. Instead of seeing things as they truly are, our past experiences, beliefs and even our moods can make us perceive things in a skewed way. And while these biases might've been super-handy for our ancestors, in today's world they can sometimes lead us up the garden path.

With confirmation bias, we cherry-pick information that snugly fits our beliefs and conveniently turns a blind eye to anything that might challenge them. Picture having a soft spot for a certain health trend. You might find yourself diving deep into success stories while breezing past the scientific evidence that shouts, 'Hold on a minute!' Or, if you've got your knickers in a twist about a particular topic, you might only spot the news that fuels your viewpoint, conveniently missing alternative facts and viewpoints. Clocking these biases in ourselves and giving them a gentle nudge can help us keep our feet firmly on the ground. Here are a few strategies for embracing uncertainty in decision-making:

1. Reframe uncertainty: Instead of seeing uncertainty as a threat, try to see it as an opportunity for learning and growth. This shift in perspective can help reduce anxiety and increase your willingness to take calculated risks.
2. Seek information: Don't overdo it, though. While there are times when information matters, those occasions are far less than you think they are. At some point, you have to accept that you've gathered enough information and it's time to make a decision.
3. Trust your intuition: Sometimes your gut instinct can guide you when logic and reason fall short.

Trust Yourself

Self-trust plays a significant role in embracing uncertainty, particularly in the context of decision-making. Self-trust is having confidence in your ability to think, make decisions and cope with the outcomes of those decisions, even when they lead to unexpected or challenging circumstances.

When you trust yourself, you believe in your ability to manage whatever comes your way, including the unknown and uncertain. This trust can help you feel more comfortable with uncertainty, because you know that, no matter what happens, you have the skills and resilience to handle it.

Self-trust can help you make choices without having complete certainty about the outcomes. You trust in your ability to make good decisions, to learn from your mistakes, and to adapt and adjust as necessary. This can make the process of decision-making less anxiety-provoking, even when there's a high degree of uncertainty involved.

Building self-trust often involves developing self-awareness, practising self-compassion and cultivating a growth mindset. It's about recognising your strengths, acknowledging your limitations and believing in your capacity to learn and grow.

Research has shown that self-trust is associated with a range of positive outcomes, including better mental health, greater resilience, and improved performance and satisfaction in various areas of life.

If It's Not a Yes, It's a No

If it's not a resounding 'Hell, yes' then it's a no. Can you let it be that simple? If you can't, then it will be invaluable to explore what your mind has to offer about the idea of doing this. Decision-making is an integral part of life; each choice shapes your path and defines your experiences. I liken indecision to sitting in the waiting room of a train station. While the world moves around you, you remain stationary, held back by fears of missing out or the possibility of failure. But by waiting, by not making a decision, you're already missing out on all the journeys and destinations life has to offer.

Every decision, whether it leads to failure or success, propels you forward. It's an opportunity to exercise your agency, to shape your life in the way you envision. So, the next time you find yourself in life's metaphorical waiting room, consider the places you could go, the experiences you could have, and take that first step towards your next journey.

Chapter 8

Criticism

Whether it's praise or criticism, you are programmed to care about what others think of you. Caring about how our actions and behaviours are perceived by those around us is an innate survival mechanism that has been ingrained in our DNA for millennia. Throughout history, our survival has depended (and still does) on the acceptance and approval of our community. Being rejected or ostracised meant being cast out from the safety and support of our community, leaving us vulnerable to the harsh realities of being alone in the world, which would almost certainly mean death. So, it's no wonder that the fear of what other people think has such a profound impact on our thoughts and actions. But as the Roman philosopher, Seneca, once said 'We suffer more often in imagination than in reality'.

However, while it's natural to seek validation and consider the opinions of others, that doesn't mean your life has to be governed by ruminating on negative thoughts. Fear of what other people will think – loved ones, colleagues and even complete strangers – often holds us back from making the moves we want to in our lives.

All You Ever Do Is Criticise

Criticism is a topic that holds a special place in my heart. It's something I've personally grappled with, been coached on a lot and have spent a significant amount of time coaching my clients on. Criticism can take various forms, both actual and perceived. It can range from venomous words aimed at tearing us down to well-intentioned feedback that our body and brain interpret as an attack. Whether it comes from others or from within ourselves, criticism has the power to deeply impact our thoughts, emotions and behaviours.

Recall the last time you felt criticised. What happened? Were you being criticised or did you interpret someone's words or actions as criticism? How did you respond? Did you take it on board in a helpful way, reject it while feeling calm and centred or did your stress response system jump into fight, flight or freeze?

If you became defensive, you might have engaged in arguments in your head or verbally defended yourself. This was the fight response, causing tension in your body and a heightened sense of readiness for conflict. If, on the other hand, your flight response was activated, you might have left the room, retreated to a toilet or attempted to hide behind your computer screen, hoping that nobody would see you. If you went into freeze mode, though, you might have sought to protect yourself by shutting down, physically and mentally withdrawing from the situation. And hopefully there are times when it's water off a duck's back, either because you know that the criticism is utterly ridiculous or because you see the value of taking it on board and using it constructively, recognising its validity and being open to it without it dismantling your sense of self.

You probably experience all the variations I've just mentioned at one time or another, or you might tend to go more in one direction. It's going to vary depending on context, too. That means the actual situation and environment that you're in, who you're with and how you interpret their behaviour (if they're on your side or not), and your level of stress prior to the conversation even starting. If you're experiencing stress, pressure or overwhelm then your survival brain is already online, making it harder to think logically and be receptive to the feedback that's helpful.

If you have a menstrual cycle, then another factor to consider is where you are in it. In the first half of the cycle, as ovulation approaches, my clients feel less challenged by feedback and more able to shut down unfair criticism, whereas when their period is due, they're more likely to want to go to battle, run away, hide and cry it out (if you don't track or work with your cycle, but you'd like to, be sure to read my previous book, *Period Power*, and head to www.maisiehill.com for my free resources to get you started). Additionally, how we respond to criticism can be influenced by various factors, such as fatigue, hunger, physical discomfort, mental health, emotional well-being and changing hormone levels during the perimenopause transition.

Being socialised as female can amplify the tendency to rely on external validation. We're usually socialised to believe that others' opinions carry more weight than our own, in turn, caring more about what others think of us rather than what we think of ourselves. From childhood through adulthood, societal conditioning encourages us to be 'good girls' and conform to expectations (I'm 42 years old and there are occasions when people insist on telling me I'm a 'good girl'). As a result, even the slightest criticism can cause our self-assurance to crumble.

Feeling Good as Hell

When we receive praise, we get a hit of dopamine – the same chemical that's released when we fall in love – and it feels fantastic. There's nothing wrong with experiencing the elation that comes from praise, you are literally designed to respond in that way and it would be ridiculous to propose or attempt to change that, but many of my clients realise that they've become overly reliant on it.

My client Sam wanted to get coached on the paralysis she was experiencing at work. She described feeling at the mercy of the feedback she received on any particular day or hour. If her work was complimented, she would feel amazing, but if she received feedback about improvements that could be made or things she had missed, it would devastate her. Sam would start thinking that her work wouldn't be good enough and that she'd be chastised by her boss in front of her colleagues. Even though her thinking brain knew that this was unlikely because she had a great boss, her survival brain was running the show. I explained that when you're very responsive to praise, you're also highly responsive to criticism and that one way to be less affected by criticism is to stop being so affected by praise.

Praise feels great and there's nothing wrong with it; we all carry a need to receive validation from others and that's not going away any time soon. But if praise can cause you to swing in one direction, then feedback and criticism will send you swaying in the opposite direction.

There's nothing wrong with being buoyed by praise, but there's a way to experience it without it becoming all you rely on. Think about it like a cake: The layers of the cake are formed by your own view of yourself (your self-concept) and the icing is the praise that comes from others. Icing by itself is delicious for a moment, but quickly becomes sickly. Cake on its own is great, but a dab of icing on a cupcake, or a smear of jam between two layers of Victoria sponge, is a beautiful thing and I'm not one to deny myself or anyone else the deliciousness of the icing on the cake. However, I suggest keeping it at that rather than using praise to prop yourself up. Don't make your emotional well-being dependent on what other people say about you. Instead, detach yourself from the emotional sway of praise.

Self-concept

Your self-concept is your internal sense of who you are – how you perceive yourself, your attributes, identities and roles, and your beliefs about what's possible for you. It also relates to self-esteem, self-awareness, self-image and self-efficacy (your belief in your capacity to do what's necessary to reach your goals).

Self-concept is developed predominantly in childhood and early adulthood when your overarching sense of who you are is more malleable and easier to update, but that doesn't mean it can't be updated later in life, it just requires a bit of effort.

Your self-concept affects your attitudes, motivations and behaviours – students who perceive themselves to be academic are more likely to achieve academic success, which in turn solidifies their beliefs.

But your self-concept isn't always congruent with reality. Every week, I coach clients whose self-concept is diminished in some way. They're more prone to putting themselves down than seeing just how fantastic and successful they are. One of the key things we work on is improving their self-concept, so that they can see what's possible for them, as opposed to what isn't. Helping them to see themselves through a more accurate lens has a positive impact on every aspect of their lives.

Criticism Versus Feedback

The line between feedback and criticism is wobbly and indistinct, so rather than trying to separate one from the other, here's how I recommend you think about it: it's simply someone offering you their opinion. It might be unsolicited and could even cross a boundary (especially if it's an opinion about your body or fertility), but it's only an opinion that, for whatever reason, they've decided to share with you.

You and I might agree that it would be great if they didn't say these things, but at the same time can we acknowledge that people make these comments because they care? Can we hold space for that duality? Our brains have a negativity bias which means we're quick to spot what isn't 'right'. When my partner does the dishes, my brain spots how they haven't been stacked 'correctly' and it feels helpful to tell him how to do it in what I perceive as the right way. When your colleague points out a mistake on a document or offers a different way of going about things, they likely think that they're being helpful, so try considering that they're on your side.

A teacher told me about a time when a student didn't like how they were being taught and threatened that their parent would come in and pull them up on it. This was a situation where they were being criticised, with the additional 'threat' of parents coming in to voice their criticism. Her response to this child was nothing short of amazing. She told them how amazing it was that they had parents who cared enough to criticise and complain, and that they should absolutely do that. Rather than get defensive, she was able to see how fortunate this kid was to have parents who cared.

What people share could feel very neutral to them, but feel loaded to you. They could well have what they perceive as your best interests at heart, yet what they tell you feels devastating and intentionally hurtful. If you're already quite critical of yourself then you're likely to perceive everything through the lens of 'I'm crap' and manage to twist helpful feedback as a criticism of your being. Even comments intended as praise somehow become faults.

Containing Criticism

Dealing with criticism can be a challenging experience, because of its ability to stir up a range of emotions and self-doubt. It can have such a huge effect that everything you were criticised for during childhood suddenly comes along for the ride when you're standing in the office having a conversation with your team leader or texting your mate.

When you're faced with criticism, it's crucial to distinguish between the specific situation at hand and the broader narrative that you construct in your mind. To do that, practise containing the psychological impact of criticism to the specific situation. Ask yourself if the criticism is truly about you as a person or if it's directed at your actions or behaviour in a particular situation. Criticism is usually more about what we did or said rather than a personal attack on our character. By recognising this distinction you can prevent the criticism from triggering a cascade of negative thoughts and spiralling into self-doubt or shame.

You also want to question if the criticism is valid and warranted. Take a step back and, as best you can, objectively evaluate the feedback. Is there any truth or constructive insight in what is being said? If so, try to separate the criticism from your sense of self-worth and acknowledge that everyone makes mistakes or has areas for improvement.

Criticism is an opportunity for growth and self-reflection rather than a reflection of your inherent value as a person. Criticism can be an opportunity to explore things in a deeper way. It brings a topic that could be a blind spot in your periphery into focus and that provides a wonderful opportunity if you're able to be open to leveraging it.

All that said, it's equally important to recognise that not all criticism is valid or fair. Sometimes people project their own insecurities or biases on to others, so their criticism may be more reflective of their own issues than your actual shortcomings. You are not defined by others' opinions or judgements. Trust in your own abilities, values and self-worth, and don't let unfounded criticism erode your self-confidence.

To effectively deal with criticism, it's helpful to practise active listening and open communication. Seek clarification and ask for specific examples to gain a deeper understanding of what's being shared. How you respond to criticism can also depend on levels of tiredness, hunger, physical pain, mental health, emotional well-being and hormone levels, because where you are in your cycle can dictate how resilient you feel and how able you are to contend with your inner critic.

Lastly, I know that not all of you exist in environments that will help you to thrive, so it's important to surround yourself with a supportive network of individuals who provide constructive feedback and encouragement. Seek out mentors, friends or colleagues who genuinely want to see you succeed and who can provide valuable insights and guidance. Their perspectives can help you navigate criticism more effectively and build resilience in the face of adversity.

Don't Let the Sound of Your Own Wheels Drive you Crazy

Rumination is defined as when you engage in an excessive, repetitive thought process that loops continuously without ever getting to a sense of completion or resolution. Rumination starts off as an attempt to problem-solve and analyse confusing or distressing situations. We replay experiences (real and imagined) to try and make sense of them and resolve them. It can also provide an opportunity to reflect on our experiences, process and understand intense emotions, and search for clarity in ambiguous and complex situations. Sounds like a great strategy, doesn't it? But it can become excessive and unproductive, ending up causing the very problems that it seeks to solve, hindering problem-solving, prolonging emotional states and contributing to the development or exacerbation of health issues.

Client Story

When Rae became a client, she was processing a recent miscarriage and facing the prospect that her husband no longer wanted to grow their family. Wondering if they were going to try again for a sibling for their eldest was never far from her thoughts: 'My mind was on rumination-repeat, over and over, unable to put to rest so many aspects from the miscarriage and what it meant for our future family planning. I was stuck on loop, and it was exhausting and took far too much mental bandwidth. Practising exquisite self-care has removed the ambiguity of how to love and support myself in the moment.

'Hearing that others are not responsible for our emotional responses was tough love, but ever so helpful. I no longer wait for my husband to understand all that the miscarriage was to me as a woman. I no longer attempt to up-skill him to get closer to understanding what my body went through. I know it's okay to release him from that responsibility and to lean on my girlfriends, who naturally can already have a much better starting point just as being women.

'I didn't know I was even speaking to myself so poorly until I started to listen and check in with myself. I hadn't had that modelled to me. I learnt how to be aware of my nervous system and how to help myself realise that I was safe. This then helped me calm down enough to address how to be kinder to myself and how to hold myself accountable to build self-trust. I am so kind in how I speak to myself. I enjoy my own company now.'

Cognitive Restructuring

Cognitive restructuring is a technique that's used in cognitive-behavioural therapy (CBT) and many coaching frameworks. It provides a way to identify and challenge unhelpful thought patterns. Here's how you can use it:

1.   Recognise what's going on. Notice if you're feeling worried or anxious, or if you're going round and round in circles in your head.
2.   Get what's in your head out of your head. The key feature of rumination is that you never get anywhere. It's the mental equivalent of being on a hamster wheel, so do something different and get off the wheel. I recommend writing your thoughts down on paper, so that you can see them for what they are.
3.   Identify negative thoughts and automatic patterns of thinking that are ingrained. Be on the lookout for cognitive distortions, such as all-or-nothing thinking, personalisation or over-generalisation (see pages 26–7).
4.   Examine these thoughts. Are they true? What factual evidence is there for them? (That doesn't mean relying on your opinion to provide facts!) What about contradictory evidence – is there any evidence that contradicts that thought?
5.   What alternative explanations and perspectives are there? Are there thoughts and beliefs that you can adopt that are adaptive and helpful?

Instead of viewing rumination purely as a pervasive thought pattern, I encourage my clients to approach it as a habit – an action they continually and, often subconsciously, take. Recognising ruminative behaviours as actions rather than abstract thought patterns can feel less daunting.

For instance, notice when you tend to ruminate most frequently. Are there particular triggers or scenarios that instigate these loops? Do these ruminative episodes correlate with certain phases in your menstrual cycle? Do they take place after spending time with a certain person, after drinking alcohol, or dropping your usual patterns of exercise? By identifying these patterns, you can actively work towards disrupting them, just as you would with any other habit.

Additionally, remember that every individual's perception is created through the lens of their personal experiences, biases and knowledge. And while it's natural to want to justify ourselves and our actions, there's a liberation in allowing people to maintain their perspective. They might not always be right about you, but you don't have to always correct them. Sometimes, the healthiest course of action is to let people be wrong about you. You don't owe everyone an explanation for who you are or the choices you make.

Instead of spiralling in the vortex of 'why don't they understand?', consider redirecting your energy. Invest it in areas where you can make real changes: your own perceptions, habits and the cultivation of self-trust. Remember that not every battle needs to be fought, and not every critic needs to be addressed. Your mental peace and well-being come first.

Chapter 9

Hard conversations

You can't go through life without encountering situations that call for difficult conversations. Discussions about unmet expectations, disagreements over decisions, or conversations about changes that need to occur can be challenging and uncomfortable, but they are also crucial for maintaining healthy relationships, understanding one another, and facilitating personal and collective growth.

We spend so much time trying to get away from what needs to be said, though. How many times have you had a conversation in your head, but held back from initiating the real conversation? While not every thought or opinion needs to be expressed out loud, avoiding conversations creates a build-up of unresolved issues, as well as strained relationships and missed opportunities for growth. It also prevents us from appreciating the perspective of others and the experience of working towards – and hopefully achieving – resolution.

Your internal world of thoughts, emotions, beliefs and fears all shape how you perceive and respond to the external world, including how you approach and navigate difficult conversations. A fear of rejection or concern about others' opinions can cause us to avoid difficult conversations in an attempt to protect ourselves from potential criticism or disapproval. If we struggle with managing uncomfortable emotions, we might shy away from conversations that could evoke these emotions, whereas developing emotional resilience can enable us to have them. And oh my goodness it is worth having them, because the more you increase your capacity for them, the greater intimacy and trust you'll have with yourself and hopefully with others too.

Fear of Others' Opinions

Some people are more practised at having hard conversations, but I don't know anyone who doesn't worry about having them or fear them in some way. And I'll be honest, no matter how skilled you get at having them, I don't think that fear ever goes away entirely, because that fear is there to serve us.

If your mind has done a great job of convincing you that you have something to fear (remembering that this can be real or imagined), then it will prevent you from having the conversation by activating your defence mechanisms. When you consider having a hard conversation, what is it that's causing you to feel this way? Is it fear of:

- Conflict
- Being yelled at
- Being reprimanded
- Rejection
- Embarrassment
- Humiliation
- Physical harm
- Standing out
- Being told you're not enough
- Being told you're too much
- Loss of the relationship or opportunity in front of you.

What does that fear tell you about the conversation? That it's important and necessary, either because it will lead to a result that you desire (like a pay rise or promotion) or because there's something that's being challenged – perhaps your boundaries, values or sense of right and wrong.

Fear is a survival mechanism that's deeply ingrained in our nature. It's designed to protect us from potential threats, be they physical, emotional or psychological. This fear isn't just limited to tangible threats; it extends to our social interactions and perceptions, particularly the fear of others' opinions. These fears can arise if you've experienced or been threatened with them in the past or because you've witnessed them happening to others in your personal and professional experiences, on social media, or in books and films.

While this fear may seem like a hindrance, it is there to serve you. Your body is on your side. The fear is simply a signal that you're venturing into potentially uncomfortable territory and your body is trying to prepare you for it, especially if the territory of uncomfortable conversations is unfamiliar to you.

Unfortunately, if this causes you to freeze, then you could find yourself unable to initiate or participate in a challenging conversation and, although you're in the room, you're not present to the conversation and are unable to articulate your thoughts or express your feelings. In fight mode, we resist the conversation by arguing against its necessity, deflecting the topic or just plain old fighting back. In flight mode, we might avoid the conversation entirely, either by physically removing ourselves from the situation or mentally distancing ourselves from the discussion.

The fawn response is another way fear can manifest. In this mode, we attempt to placate or appease the perceived threat, which in this case is the potential negative reaction of the other person. This could involve carefully crafting our words to avoid upsetting the other party; skirting around the main issue rather than addressing it directly; going along with their perspective when you don't agree with it; and unnecessarily apologising.

Stay With Me

Conversations that are challenging, confronting and stressful can also cause an individual to disassociate – a phenomenon where you feel disconnected from your thoughts, feelings, memories, body, sense of identity, or the world around you. This can manifest as a feeling of spacing out, losing track of time, or feeling detached from your body or surroundings. Disassociation is part of the human experience and everyday experiences of it include becoming so absorbed in a book or your phone that you lose awareness of what's going on around you or zoning out when driving a familiar route. It's also a defence mechanism that the brain uses to protect us from intense emotional distress and traumatic events.

Disassociation can prevent us from fully engaging in the conversation, expressing our thoughts and feelings, and both hearing and understanding the other person's perspective. In the early years of my relationship, any time my partner and I would have a remotely confrontational chat, I would forget what we were talking about in the middle of the conversation and need to ask him what it was. This was before I learned how to stay in the conversation, using grounding somatic techniques to help me reconnect with my body and physical environment.

Whether you experience disassociation or not, here are a few techniques that you can try to anchor you in the present moment. Some of them you'll be able to use during conversations, others you might prefer to use afterwards, depending on whom the conversation is with and your relationship to them, as well as the environment that you're in:

- 5-4-3-2-1 grounding technique: A personal favourite of mine, this technique engages your five senses to help you stay present. Identify five things you can see, four things you can touch, three things you can hear, two things you can smell and one thing you can taste.
- Pick a colour: Look around you and see how many items you can find in your chosen colour in your environment. This focusing technique helps you orient to your environment.
- Hug yourself: There are times when we all need to feel the safety that comes from being held and contained in a hug, and although it might sound odd at first, hugging yourself is effective.
- Wiggle your fingers and toes: This simple mindful movement exercise creates sensation in your body that helps you to connect with yourself and brings some movement into the body, which helps when you're in a freeze response. It's also very subtle, making it a great option if you don't want anyone else to notice.
- Squeezing: Gently squeeze your fists together and release them, playing with the amount of pressure as well as the tempo. You can also pinch your thumb and forefinger together. The squeezing technique is another one that you can do that will go undetected by others.
- Cupping: Cup your hand as if you were trying to hold some water in it. Softly holding this cup shape, tap all over your body to help you feel grounded and remind you of your boundaries and where you end, helping you to feel contained.
- Body scan: Close your eyes and mentally scan your body from head to toe. Do you notice any sensations, tensions or discomfort? This can help you reconnect with your physical presence.
- Progressive muscle relaxation: Similar to the body scan, this technique involves tensing and relaxing different muscle groups in your body, starting from your toes and working your way up to your head. This helps to release physical tension and bring your focus back to your body.
- Regulating resources: See pages 57–9.

Remember that it's normal to struggle with staying present during confronting conversations. Don't judge or criticise yourself if you find your mind wandering or if you start to disassociate. Instead, be gentle with yourself and guide your attention back to the present using these techniques. With practice, you'll find it easier to stay present and engaged, even during challenging discussions.

It's natural to worry about and fear difficult conversations, but rather than letting that block you from taking any action, try to see it as a necessary first step that you just need to get on the other side of. Rather than aiming to remove any and all fear, my suggestion is to be able to experience that fear and move through it. With practice and patience, it'll become increasingly straightforward.

Building Emotional Resilience

Emotional resilience is essential when it comes to navigating challenging conversations. Your ability to adapt and bounce back in the face of emotional distress, adversity or significant sources of stress can be the difference between productive dialogue and escalating conflict.

A large part of this is being able to feel your emotions, especially those that are uncomfortable, without becoming overwhelmed or reactive. It involves acknowledging and accepting your feelings, rather than avoiding or suppressing them. This ability is particularly important in challenging conversations that can evoke strong emotional responses. But this doesn't mean that you should seek to exist in a Zen-like state, completely unflustered by anything, because that would likely involve suppression of emotions, too.

Being able to feel any emotion allows you to stay present and engaged in the conversation, even when it becomes difficult. It's a way for you to honour your thoughts and feelings, while also being able to respond thoughtfully and constructively, rather than reacting impulsively or defensively.

Do You Really Want to Hurt Me?

Being honest with someone about what is or isn't working, or about what you want or don't want, involves risk – risk of being disliked, disagreed with or disapproved of. It involves being honest with yourself and with others. It requires you to put yourself out there. And with that comes the potential for rejection.

Experiencing rejection doesn't mean that you have been rejected. It might *feel* like you've been rejected, and you might *think* that you have, but that doesn't mean that you have been rejected. If that's twisting your brain in knots, I understand, but rejection isn't as black and white as we think it is. Rather than recalling a time when you experienced rejection, think about the times when you haven't replied to someone's text or email, when you forgot your brother's birthday (sorry, Sam, for doing this every year) or to invite a friend to an event. Did you purposely reject that person? On some occasions, perhaps, but overall, probably not. That won't have stopped them from potentially feeling rejected, though.

Client Story

My client Lo had been coaching herself using the framework that I teach all my clients. Lo had used it to explore her experiences of dating and specifically about how pleasing-people habits showed up when she was on dates. She noticed that she would edit herself a little bit here and a little bit there to try and be more acceptable, likeable, attractive and, ultimately, loveable. On dates, she would often censor herself and, as I coached her, she realised that this stemmed from a belief that she needed to be who they wanted her to be to avoid being rejected, which was an experience she feared, because, as we've said, it feels like crap. As a result, she ended up not being herself and not connecting with the people that she was on dates with. She had already done an amazing job of uncovering all of this for herself using the self-coaching method that I teach my clients, but I pointed out that as a result of this pattern, three things were happening:

1. She was experiencing rejection ahead of time, which happens so often with all sorts of emotions – she didn't want to experience an emotion, so she was trying to avoid it by altering her behaviour, but all that happened was she was experiencing it in her imagination anyway.
2. In trying to avoid being rejected by someone, she edited her words, behaviour and posture to be 'acceptable' and 'desirable'. Lo stopped being herself, and in doing so, rejecting herself.
3. She wasn't giving the other person a chance to accept her, because she wasn't being herself around them. She was giving them this other version of herself.

What was happening to Lo happens to lots of us to varying degrees, but, of course, the whole time that this is going on, you're also deepening the belief that you aren't acceptable or lovable as you are. Think about what that does to your relationship with yourself. It's pretty awful, isn't it?

Fear of rejection is crippling and it costs us so much. It's not exclusive to dating, so think about where fear of rejection shows up in your life. Does it appear at work, meeting with prospective/current clients, when meeting your partner's family or friends of friends, or ordering a coffee in a café? You can use what I'm sharing here to understand and bring awareness to any kind of situation where fear of rejection crops up.

It's also likely to appear any time you do something that is slightly out of the ordinary for you in some way. Anything that you think will draw attention to you will probably make you worry about being rejected on some level. If that happens to you, it's very understandable and it's just your body trying to keep you safe (even when most of the time, that's not actually true). You don't have to make it mean anything when it happens. You can just think of it as step one in the process and then move on to whatever step two looks like for you.

There's a good reason why it's so triggering to feel left out, ignored or rejected, and that's because it's painful. Rejection hurts. Researchers simulated the experience of rejection by asking people who had recently experienced an unwanted breakup to look at a photograph of their ex-partner. They then asked them to think about being rejected, all while they were having an MRI scan of their brain. They saw areas of the brain that support the sensory components of physical pain become active when they were thinking about their ex-partner and being rejected. Rejection quite literally hurts and the experience is comparable to the level of physical pain that would have you reaching for painkillers like ibuprofen or paracetamol.

Feeling awful because of rejection serves a purpose. These days, food and dwellings are far easier to come by than they were in our evolutionary past, and we don't need to rely on being part of a community to be fed and protected (though during the pandemic I think we all realised just how necessary community and mutual aid is). However, back when our survival really was dependent on being in a group it helped to have mechanisms in place to help ensure that we stayed part of the group, because if we were rejected, we'd have been kicked out of that community and had to fend for ourselves, rather than benefiting from the safety and sharing of resources and skills that comes from being in a group. Experiencing the pain of social rejection makes us more inclined to make decisions to share our resources, which in turn helps to ensure our safety and place within a group, which is what has kept us alive historically.

A Pathway to Self-acceptance

Any time you have an idea, a goal, a dream or a desire to create something, fear of rejection will emerge somehow. It's just how we're wired. This means that in order to lean into doing whatever it is that you want to do, you will have to risk dislike, disapproval and perhaps even haters. That doesn't mean it will happen – it may not be likely at all – but internally on some level you're probably convinced that it will.

If you can create a felt sense of safety within yourself, enough to take that risk, then you will simultaneously approve of yourself – the opposite of self-rejection. And then you won't need other people to approve of you so much, because you will approve, validate and accept yourself.

This shift in mindset is transformative. It can free you from the paralysing grip of fear, allowing you to pursue your goals and dreams with confidence and resilience. It can enable you to show up authentically in your work, your relationships and your life.

But let's be real. It doesn't matter what you do or don't do, some people just won't be into you or what you do. And that's perfectly okay. We're so used to worrying about what other people think of us that we fail to consider that there are plenty of people for whom you just aren't their cup of tea – that doesn't make them or you a bad person. There are also plenty of people for whom you are their cup of tea. I said this in my second book, *Perimenopause Power*, but I think it's worth repeating here – a jar of Marmite doesn't worry about the people who can't stand it and nor should you!

If you were to go to the lengths required for everyone else to like you, the other people who *are* your people won't like you. Not to mention the enormous amount of time and energy that goes into thinking about those people, let alone behaving in the way that you think they want you to, which may or may not be accurate anyway.

Trying to please everyone is not only exhausting and unfeasible, but it can also alienate the people who truly appreciate you for who you are. There will always be people who love and value you exactly as you are. So, think about your life and your goals. Are you ready to accept and love yourself?

Are you willing to risk rejection from others in order to get there? Because although other people can 'reject you' in terms of them saying or doing something, you don't have to feel rejected. You don't have to feel rejection. That's optional. It's possible for you to experience a rejection without feeling like you have been rejected.

The only reason you would feel rejected is because you think thoughts that generate the emotion of feeling rejected, because there will be times in your life, I am sure, when you have been told no and you didn't feel rejected – you were just told no and you didn't make it mean anything about you.

In the end, the path to meeting your goals lies in self-acceptance. If you continue to reject yourself, it's going to take a long time to achieve those goals or you never will. Besides, people think about you far less than you think they do. They're also unlikely to think of you in the negative ways that you think of yourself to the extent that you do.

When It Hurts So Bad

We've established that rejection doesn't feel good, but some experts suspect that it is an even more intense experience for some individuals. Rejection sensitive dysphoria (RSD) is a term that some experts use to describe those who have an overwhelming experience of emotional pain when they feel rejected, criticised or disapproved of. As it isn't an officially recognised symptom or diagnosis, there isn't much research around it (and some dispute and deny its existence), but it appears to be more common in those with ADHD (attention deficit hyperactivity disorder) brains. Those with RSD may be perceived by others as overly sensitive, perfectionist and overly reactive to even the gentlest feedback or slight criticism. *Psychology Today* highlights that because it doesn't 'officially' exist as a condition, there is no quantifiable criteria that can be used to establish if an individual has RSD or not, though they do propose that the following be used as guidance:

- High sensitivity about the possibility of rejection
- Overly high standards for yourself
- Feeling easily triggered towards guilt or shame

- Isolating yourself in a pre-emptive strike not to be rejected
- Aggressive behaviour towards those who you perceive have slighted you
- Uncomfortable physical reactions due to 'not fitting in' or being misunderstood
- Self-esteem that is entirely dependent on what others think, and rises and falls accordingly
- Frequent and intense ruminating after an interaction about how you did or said something wrong.

This is ongoing work for me, particularly as I'm autistic. Sensitivity to criticism is an autistic trait and it's common for autistic people to be very hard on themselves, in addition to experiences of criticism and rejection for being 'different'. Loved ones can ask me the simplest of questions and there's a part of me that jumps into defending myself. Most of the time there's really no need for it, but I no longer judge myself for it, because for most of my life I have felt like an outsider, and there have been many times when I've been misunderstood and that's led to threatening behaviour from others. So, I have learned to appreciate that my missiles are getting ready to launch and understand why, while also reassuring myself that they're not actually needed. I am good with me being me and I have my own back, no matter what.

Mindset Matters

Our thoughts play a significant role in shaping our actions, particularly when it comes to initiating or participating in important conversations. Often, it's not the conversation itself that hinders us, but our thoughts and beliefs about it. These thoughts can create a sense of apprehension and discomfort, leading us to avoid or withdraw from potentially challenging discussions and even straightforward or delightful ones.

These beliefs often serve as defence mechanisms, attempting to shield us from potential discomfort. However, they can also prevent us from addressing important issues, expressing our feelings or fostering deeper connections with others. By identifying and challenging these beliefs, we can begin to dismantle the barriers they create, paving the way for more open, honest and productive conversations. Let's knock them down, one by one.

It's going to be hard/stressful

Yes, it probably will be. So what? You're already experiencing stress by having it in your head, so you may as well have it out loud. What are the benefits to you doing it, even if it's hard, stressful and feels awful? What might your next experience of a hard conversation be like if you're willing to have this one now? And what about the one after that? Imagine committing to having one hard conversation a week – telling your sister that you won't be going to your niece's sixth birthday party, talking to your boss about a pay rise and sending your food back because the restaurant got your order wrong. Within a month you'll create a new neural pathway, and an entirely different level of belief and trust in yourself. You can also find some other, more helpful ways of thinking about the conversation. I don't recommend swapping 'It's going to be hard' for 'It's going to be easy' unless you believe it will be, but can you find a sentence that both acknowledges how you currently feel *and* creates space for it to go well? Try these on for size:

- 'This will probably go better than I anticipate' (particularly useful if you're prone to thinking that the worst will happen).
- 'It will be a relief to be on the other side of this conversation' (because you'll know either way and the brain loves certainty).
- 'They are not the enemy' (I use this one a lot when I need to remind myself that Paul and I are on the same team).

I'll disappoint them

That's a strong possibility. You are going to disappoint some people, but that doesn't make you disappointing, you're just not doing what they want you to do. And so what if someone is disappointed in your decision? What will happen? Get your brain to answer this question, because unless you interrogate this idea, it will keep things vague and the fear of disappointing someone will loom around. If the other person is disappointed, what are they likely to do? Will they make a face, sigh, shake their head or text you to express their disappointment? Once you're more specific, ask yourself if it's in your capability to handle it.

I'll make them angry

That could happen too. And then what? What does your brain think they will do if they're angry? Will they yell at you, will they hit you, or will they huff and puff and shut a cupboard door slightly louder than usual? It's good to know these things, because sometimes our brains go to the most dramatic places and that's always in service of your survival. Of course, it may also be because of previous experiences of verbal and/or physical abuse (or witnessing others having that experience).

There's no point talking about it

Clearly there is or you would have let go of the idea of doing it. So, are you just deciding it will result in a crappy outcome to get out of doing it?

I don't know what to say

Telling yourself 'I don't know what to say' is an understandable thought, but I'm 99.99 per cent sure that it isn't true. Here's why: if we could wave a magic wand and, no matter what you said to this person, they smiled and wholeheartedly agreed with you, would you know what to say? When I ask my clients to remove all potential threats and instead imagine that whatever words come out of their mouth will be received in the best of ways, they find that they do know what to say. What's been holding them back is fear that something negative will happen, so they've been searching for the perfect words that will result in zero conflict or discomfort.

Once you know what it is that you want to say, check to see if it aligns with what you want the conversation to result in. You might think that these things are one and the same, but they aren't.

The Worst-case Scenario

When faced with the prospect of a difficult conversation, it's natural for your mind to jump to the worst-case scenario. What if the other person is disappointed or angry with your decision? What if they express their disappointment or anger towards you? These questions can create a sense of dread and anxiety, making the conversation seem even more daunting.

When my clients first start working with me, many of them try to avoid thinking about the worst-case scenario, because, well, let's face it, it doesn't feel good and on some level they're usually aware that where their mind is going is unlikely to happen. However, while there are times when we can steer our brain away from these thought patterns, it can be helpful to explore these worst-case scenarios in detail. By using the 'and then what?' technique from page 152, you can explore what it is that you're really worried about.

For example, if someone is disappointed in your decision, they might express their disappointment to you. And then what? You might feel sad, annoyed, guilty or even ashamed. As you continue this line of questioning, you'll likely find that the ultimate fear is not the reaction of the other person, but the emotion that you'll experience as a result. The result of this chain of events is that you feel an emotion. This realisation can be incredibly liberating, because emotions, while powerful, are also manageable. And if you know that you're capable of feeling any emotion, then the fear of the worst-case scenario loses a lot of its power. Yes, you might feel sad, annoyed, guilty or ashamed, but you've felt these emotions before and you've survived. You've learned from them, grown from them and moved forward, and you will this time too. Reaching this place often helps you to see that, even in the worst of times, you still have options and you will know what to do.

So, the next time you're dreading a difficult conversation, ask yourself, 'And then what?' and keep asking until you've reached the end of the scenario. Then remind yourself that whatever emotion you might feel, you can handle it. This can help to alleviate some of the heaviness and fear surrounding the conversation, allowing you to approach it with more confidence and clarity.

How to Have a Constructive Conversation

Navigating challenging conversations is an art that requires both empathy and strategy. While the mere thought of initiating such discussions can be intimidating, being equipped with some techniques can make a world of difference. Not only can these strategies alleviate some of the apprehension you might feel, but they can also pave the way for a more constructive and fruitful dialogue. Here are some techniques I recommend using to make facing difficult conversations less daunting and ensure the conversation itself is more productive.

Focus on the desired outcome

This sounds obvious and simple, but it's where you're most likely to get tripped up, because to do this you'll need to care more about your future than your past, and brains love nothing more than reverting to the past hurts and injustices.

Thinking in advance about what a good outcome could look like is important, because your thinking brain is more likely to be engaged than in the heat of the moment, making it easier to be solution focused. Whereas if your stress response system is engaged then your survival brain will have you focused on protecting and defending yourself. It's also worth thinking about what happens if you end up with your desired outcome, and what happens if you don't.

The goal isn't to be able to have every conversation like a robot. It's to mobilise use of your defence mechanisms when it's appropriate to, and to disarm your missile defence system when it's not needed. I can't tell you when you should do what – that's for you to discern and experiment with, and experimentation involves failure, so you won't always get it right, whatever right is. But remember that relationships are built on the experience of going through ruptures and repairs.

All Apologies

If the outcome you want is for someone to apologise, let's imagine that they do – what will that give you and how will you feel? Is that feeling available to you now, without requiring them to behave a certain way? Because although you might want an apology from someone, that doesn't mean that you're going to get one and I don't recommend making your ability to get to a place of closure dependent on someone else. For a start, they may not want to have the conversation, and there's a strong chance that they won't say the exact words that you want them to say in the exact tone and manner that you want them to. And it's okay for you to want that, truly, but expecting people to be different than they are is a recipe for hurt and disaster.

There are times when someone is clueless and on hearing that they've messed something up, they do offer an authentic apology of their own accord, but I personally have no interest in receiving an apology that I've demanded from someone, because their words are meaningless. I would rather focus on expressing myself honestly and explicitly to them, and being open to whatever happens next. Entering a conversation with 'I need you to apologise' may result in you getting what you want in the short term, but with negative consequences in the long term, because how does it feel when someone is forced into apologising? Does it create more connection or less?

Be ready for ruptures and repairs

Ruptures, or conflicts, in relationships can feel distressing and uncomfortable, leading many of us to avoid them whenever possible. This is particularly true for those who haven't had much experience with healthy conflicts and healing repairs. If these weren't modelled for you growing up, the concept might feel foreign and intimidating, but ruptures are a natural part of human relationships and they don't necessarily signify something negative about you, the other person or your relationship. In fact, experiencing ruptures and working through them can strengthen relationships. The more evidence you gather that it's okay to have disagreements and then repair the relationship, the more comfortable you'll become with this process. Over time, the experience of conflict won't feel as severe or threatening.

In every verbal and non-verbal communication that you have with someone else, your nervous system is interacting with their nervous system. Both of you are running that software in the background that's always on the lookout for potential threats and safety cues. If you can start viewing every interaction through this lens, you will radically shift your experience of your personal and professional relationships.

However, when you do this, focus on your own reactions and behaviours rather than trying to analyse or diagnose the other person's. I really don't recommend that you tell the people in your life about themselves if someone is in a heightened emotional state or behaving in a way that suggests their fight-or-flight response has been triggered. They probably don't want you telling them how they feel! Instead, stay in your own lane and mind your own business. If you find yourself focusing more on their behaviour than your own, this could be a defence mechanism.

You can't control how others react, but you can control your own responses. This will allow you to navigate ruptures more effectively and contribute to the repair process in a constructive and empathetic way. Successful ruptures and repairs are an opportunity for growth, understanding and deepening connection. By understanding your own reactions and focusing on your own behaviour, you can navigate these conflicts in a more productive way.

Acknowledge the issue

This can be as simple as saying, 'I think there's something we need to discuss,' or 'I've noticed that we've been avoiding this topic.' Express your thoughts and feelings honestly, but respectfully. Use 'I' statements to express your perspective without blaming or criticising others. How can you have this conversation while being 100 per cent responsible for yourself?

Listen

A lot of this chapter is about how to speak up and that is important, but so too is listening. Give others the opportunity to express their thoughts and feelings without interrupting. Extend to them the same respect you want to receive from them. As you listen, try to find areas of common ground and the places where you agree.

Avoid the tit-for-tat trap

One of the common pitfalls in any challenging conversation is falling into the tit-for-tat trap and I have no doubt that you've experienced it – the conversation escalates into a back-and-forth exchange of accusations and counter-accusations, with past mistakes and perceived injustices all being dredged up. Before you know it, you've lost the point of the conversation, and only increased defensiveness and disconnection. This approach rarely leads to a productive outcome and can significantly strain the relationship.

If you want to improve your communication in a relationship, decide that you won't do this (even if the other person does). Instead of getting into 'You did this' and 'Yeah, but what about this thing that you did?', stay focused on the outcome you want to create. This means being more committed to the future than the past. Instead of clinging to your sense of justice or the overwhelming urge to be right (and oh my days, believe me when I say how familiar I am with that urge!), concentrate on what you want to achieve from the conversation. This could be a resolution to a specific problem, a deeper understanding of each other's perspectives or an improvement in your relationship.

This will require you to consciously de-arm your missile defence system, which is quite something when you feel threatened or as if you're under attack (or at least a part of you believes that you are). Seek to understand rather than win. Approach the conversation with the goal of understanding the other person's perspective, not to win the argument or prove them wrong.

Make requests, not demands

I don't know a single person who relishes demands being made of them. It's something that we all resist and buck against, and yet we're very good at being demanding of others ourselves. In the context of relationships and challenging conversations, understanding the difference between requests and demands is crucial. Both are forms of communication expressing a desire or need, but they differ significantly in their implications, tone and potential outcomes.

Requests are respectful and considerate expressions of one's needs or desires. They are open-ended and allow for the possibility of a 'no' without negative repercussions. When you make a request, you acknowledge the other person's autonomy and right to choose their response. This fosters a sense of mutual respect and understanding, which can facilitate more productive and less confrontational conversations. For example, a request might be, 'Could we discuss our financial situation this evening? I think it's important for us to be on the same page.'

Demands, on the other hand, are more forceful and directive. They imply an expectation of compliance and often carry an underlying threat of consequences if not met. Demands can create a power imbalance in the relationship and often lead to defensiveness or resistance, which can escalate into conflict and ultimatums. An example of a demand might be, 'We are discussing our finances tonight, whether you like it or not.'

If you're not in the practice of making requests, then beginning to ask for things could feel momentous and like it's a really big deal. For most of my clients, the requests that they're making aren't exactly extravagant, but that doesn't stop those requests from feeling huge to them.

In challenging conversations, it's generally more effective to use requests rather than demands. Requests encourage open dialogue, mutual respect and collaborative problem-solving. They allow both parties to express their needs and perspectives without feeling threatened or coerced – something I think we can all agree is preferable.

Tone, body language and context can significantly influence how a request or demand is perceived. Even a request can come across as a demand if delivered in a harsh tone or accompanied by negative body language. So, it's not just what you say, but how you say it.

Pick your time and place

Even when you make a request can make a difference. Timing is a crucial yet often overlooked aspect of effective communication. When the other person is already stressed or preoccupied, they are less likely to be able to fully engage in the conversation. If someone's had a tricky day at work or a deadline is looming, their capacity to listen, understand and respond thoughtfully can be significantly diminished. They may be more prone to react defensively or dismissively, which can escalate the conflict and hinder resolution.

While it can be useful to consider the other person's state of mind and current circumstances before initiating a difficult conversation, you don't need to swing all the way in the other direction and end up dismissing your own needs, choosing a time when they are likely to be more relaxed and receptive, but you won't be.

If an issue needs to be addressed immediately, it may not be possible to wait for the perfect time (not that it even exists). In these cases, acknowledging the less-than-ideal timing can help. For example, you might say, 'I realise this might not be the best time, but this is an important issue that I think we need to address.'

While there can be more opportune times than others, for most people there's always something going on, and I don't think it's useful to save up and store all your important conversations for holidays. The ideal is that you get to the point where you're able to talk about these things casually and on an ongoing basis.

Where you talk can also greatly influence the conversation. As experienced as I am with managing my mind and tending to my nervous system, having an important conversation while I'm walking around (either side by side or with someone on the phone) is always going to be a more positive experience than sitting opposite each other at a table or communicating through a device. Talking while doing a menial task also seems to take the heat and intensity out of things, because it gives my body something to do, which means I'm less likely to go into fight, flight or freeze. If you're able to, have conversations in environments that are supportive for you, the other person and your conversation.

Account for stress levels and responses

Your own stress levels can create a sense of urgency that significantly interferes with productive conversations by impairing your ability to think clearly, make rational decisions and consider the other person's perspective. You might be more prone to making snap judgements or jumping to conclusions without fully understanding the situation (hey, we've all been there).

When you're stressed, you're more likely to become defensive or to react emotionally to what's being said, making it harder to have a calm and respectful conversation. Stress can also distract you from truly listening to the other person. You can become more focused on your own thoughts, feelings or what you're going to say next, preventing you from fully hearing and understanding the other person's perspective. And if your stress levels create a sense of urgency, you might rush the conversation, not giving it the time and attention it deserves. This, combined with an impaired ability to listen to others, can lead to misunderstandings and missed information. It can also put pressure on the other person, making them feel rushed or stressed themselves. And although there may be times when you wish to impart a sense of urgency to others, it usually creates a tense environment that's not conducive to open and honest communication.

Clearly, it's important to manage your sense of urgency. While some conversations will be urgent, I recommend pausing and asking yourself if it's true that they are, and to do what you can to ensure that any urgency doesn't compromise the quality or outcome of the conversation. If you're both already feeling stressed, then it might not take much for your missiles to become activated or to initiate an escape plan. If you can have a conversation while also observing and tending to your nervous system, then your capacity for doing so will grow and you'll gradually build the skill of being able to stay in the conversation.

Without doubt, there will be times when you feel the need to defend yourself or escape – and that's okay. Remember the goal isn't to suppress these responses, it's to be able to work within them and give yourself options. Do you want to yell at your dad for doing something you're not happy about? I'm here for it, but if your sense is that your missile system is being activated in an unhelpful way, then you might decide you want to work on responding differently.

If a colleague has a knack of dismissing your contributions and you tend to freeze or shut down in some way, then it might be useful to work on letting yourself get activated and bringing those defence mechanisms online. If people-pleasing or retreating has been your go-to way of reacting, or if growing up, anger and the behaviours associated with it were frowned on or resulted in punishment, then getting defensive might feel risky or even dangerous. That can be because there are internal beliefs for you to unwind or because you're not used to feeling so much activation within you.

There is no one right way to respond in any situation, which is why I can't give you a prescriptive solution and, even if I could, it's more important that you develop your own internal guidance system and learn to trust yourself. There are times when you'll fuck it up, but everything else in this book will help you to be okay with that. Besides, each fuck up gives you an opportunity to practise and experience repairs.

Plan For When Things Feel Too Much

Those are ideas for techniques that will help you have more constructive conversations, but what about when you or they simply need to walk away? Well, sometimes that is the best thing, but can you honour that while also creating some space for connection (if that's what you want)? Here are some suggestions for what you might have ready to say when it all gets a bit overwhelming:

- This is important for us to discuss but I need to take a break, so that I can take care of my nervous system and take on board what you're saying.
- We've covered a lot and I'd like to really take on board what you've said, so how about we take a break and then check in later today/this week, so that we can resolve things?
- I care about you/this conversation and it feels like the best way to take care of myself so that we can continue in a productive way with it is to take some space, so I'm going to move my body/take a bath etc. Can we see how we're both doing after that?

Chapter 10

Self-responsibility

I'm about to convince you that taking responsibility is one of the most empowering things you can do for your life. I get it if you're a bit wary about the idea of being responsible. After all, dictionary definitions like 'to blame someone or something' and 'to be the person who caused something to happen, especially something bad' can make the concept seem less than appealing. But let's flip the script for a moment. What if you were the one responsible for something going well? Wouldn't you want to be credited for a success?

We're all quick to accept the credit when things go well, but when things go awry we're often less eager to step up. This is where the concept of self-responsibility comes in. It's about recognising that you are the primary cause of your experiences and, therefore, you can be credited or blamed for them.

When my clients first become members of Powerful, they often exhibit patterns of over-responsibility in some areas of their life and under-responsibility in others. Trust me, I've been there too, because as humans we tend to hang out in extremes. We're prone to all-or-nothing thinking and behaviour, and this applies to responsibility too. We either swing in one direction, taking on far too much responsibility for things that aren't ours to manage, or we swing in the other direction, shirking responsibility for things that are within our control. While neither of these extremes feel great, they might feel comfortable because they're familiar.

Over-responsibility can leave you feeling consumed with stress and worry, because you're over-functioning for others. Under-responsibility, on the other hand, can leave you feeling detached and disconnected, and result in you blaming others and the circumstances of your life. Self-responsibility, however, feels solid, grounded and powerful. You won't carry the weight that comes from over-functioning, nor will you fall into victim mode by making everyone else responsible for how you feel and blaming others (or yourself).

Blame implies that someone is at fault and, let's be honest, it doesn't feel good. It's disempowering. If you're blaming someone else, you're making them responsible for your life. Can you see how disempowering that is? Blaming, judging and berating yourself produces a whole host of negative feelings: shame, humiliation, self-pity... the list goes on. So, of course, your brain will resist taking responsibility if it associates it with these negative emotions, but this isn't being self-responsible, it's getting caught in the blame and shame cycle, and that's completely different.

Hot Potato

Accountability and blame are words that get tossed around and lumped together, but they are fundamentally different. Blame is the act of pointing fingers, assigning fault and accusing ourselves or others when things go wrong. It's a reactive stance that often leads to feelings of shame, guilt and resentment. It's like a hot potato that no one wants to hold, so it gets thrown around and causes more harm than good.

Accountability is a proactive approach that involves taking ownership of our actions, decisions and their consequences. When we're accountable, we're not looking for faults or scapegoats. Instead of being paralysed with shame, we're able to productively assess and reflect on our limitations and mishaps, while seeking understanding and benefitting from learning opportunities. We're able to reflect on our actions and decisions, assess their impacts and make necessary adjustments. This process empowers us to grow and evolve.

Now, let's talk about responsibility. Responsibility is the commitment to carry out our duties and obligations. When we're responsible, we ensure that we're doing our part, fulfilling our roles and meeting our commitments to ourselves, others and our long-term goals.

It's Not Them, It's You

It's oh-so-tempting to blame circumstances or other people for our personal feelings – we all do it. Pointing our fingers at external factors – time, technology, the weather, your hormones, the buses – blaming them for our behaviour and making them responsible for our emotional state. This blame game, however, is a clear sign of abdicating responsibility. It's a way of making others or external factors responsible for our emotional well-being, which is, in fact, our own responsibility.

Imagine you have a meeting scheduled for 9 a.m. You wake up late, get stuck in traffic and arrive at the meeting 30 minutes late. If you're being under-responsible, you might shrug it off and not take any ownership of the situation. You might say, 'Well, it's not my fault that the traffic was bad,' or 'My phone ran out of battery so the alarm didn't go off.' While these statements might be true, they're also a form of denial, where you're blaming external circumstances and avoiding taking responsibility for your actions and their consequences.

If you're self-responsible, you would acknowledge your involvement in the situation. You might say, 'I could have plugged my phone in,' or' I could have checked the traffic before leaving.' This is a form of accountability, where you're recognising your role and thinking about how you could prevent it from happening again in the future. It doesn't necessarily mean saying these things to others. It can, but what's most important is being honest with yourself.

The key difference here is that under-responsibility and blaming external factors both avoid taking ownership of what happened, while self-responsibility acknowledges your part in it. When something undesirable happens, try observing what's taken place from a neutral position. Instead of jumping into blame, guilt and shame, get curious and understand your role in the situation. This is the essence of self-responsibility.

Carrying the World

People who are over-responsible are very good at responding to the needs of others, often not needing to be asked to do things, because they're so adept at anticipating them in advance. They tend to be pretty crap at asking for help and receiving help that's offered, and as a result have very busy schedules, ones where their own priorities and pursuits get demoted at the first whiff of being needed or wanted elsewhere. Though they may smile (genuinely or insincerely) on the outside, sadness and resentment are usually simmering and accumulating on the inside, or they feel a strong sense of guilt when they take any time for themselves.

Over-responsibility is a common trait that many of us carry, often without realising it. It's the tendency to take on more than what is reasonably ours to handle. It can stem from various factors: If you grew up in an environment where caregivers were unable to adequately fulfil their responsibilities, you might have needed to step in and take on those duties, and ended up being more parent than child. Or you got the sense that your needs didn't matter; that there was no space for them. You might have been the eldest child in the family or one of many children. Maybe you had a sibling who was ill or who had things going on that resulted in them getting what we could call 'attention' or 'taking up resources', whether that was time, money or love, and so you were rewarded for not making a fuss and for being helpful. There might have been an air of 'Thank goodness we don't have to worry about you – you're so helpful, understanding, and sensible.' Maybe your school reports described you in that way, too.

Another characteristic of over-responsibility is the tendency to seek validation through helping others. This can lead to resentment when the help given is not sufficiently acknowledged or appreciated. There's nothing wrong with helping others; it's when we do so with the expectation of receiving praise or bolstering our identity that it becomes problematic.

Over-responsibility can also be linked to people-pleasing behaviours. People-pleasers often suppress their own needs and desires to avoid conflict and negative emotions. They respond to the demands and expectations of others, sometimes even to unspoken ones, and feel guilty if they don't fulfil these perceived obligations.

In the professional realm, over-responsibility can lead to burnout, as individuals may take on more tasks than they can handle, often out of a desire to be seen as reliable or indispensable, but resulting in a lack of work-life balance and increased stress levels.

Client Story

My client Roxy has experienced burnout and here she describes how understanding stress responses has helped her recover from that and change her perspective on life:

'I was a very bright and curious kid, who always did well in school. I was extremely shy, though, and didn't know how to ask for help. I felt like I had to figure everything out by myself and be the 'easy one'. My parents were always very supportive of anything I did and didn't put pressure on me to succeed, but my father was mostly absent and my mother emotionally volatile sometimes.

'She had a full plate with me, my hyperactive twin brothers and my often-absent father. She was often ill and overwhelmed, and didn't get to carve out her own life until after we grew up. She had war-traumatised and narcissistic parents who never taught her safety and how to regulate her emotions. She made us feel unconditionally loved (something she never had), but created an unsafe environment in which sometimes our struggles and feelings would be met with anger and aggression. So I learned to make myself small and shy, the self-reliant "good girl", who was actually very dependent on her praise and affection.

'Learning about the nervous system made me understand where my mother's outbursts came from and helped me to identify my own "shutdown" state. I experienced pretty severe burnout working on my PhD and coaching helped me to see which thought/feeling patterns and stress states had led me there. Over the course of my membership [of Powerful] I've worked on a very radical shift in the way I talk to myself and how I look at life.

'I have much more understanding and compassion about where I am and how far I've come. I've cultivated self-love and self-trust, and am decoupling my self-worth from performance and achievements (of course, it's all a work-in-progress but that's okay). I can recognise and manage when I feel stressed or shut-down, and honour what I need in that moment. I have developed a vision for the near future and I trust I can realise it, even though it is bolder than I've ever dreamed and I'm not fully healed from burnout.

'One of Maisie's phrases I think about a lot is "What if you did know what to do?" She also says, "What if you just decide?" and I find it's true. I have the wisdom I need to take care of myself.'

Martyr Mums

Growing up with a parent who embodies the role of a martyr can significantly shape your perspective on responsibility and self-worth. Often, these parents – typically mums – are overly responsible, taking on more than their fair share of duties and obligations, and sacrificing their own needs and desires for the sake of others.

This behaviour is usually driven by a deep-seated need for validation and a fear of being seen as selfish or uncaring. When somebody doesn't receive the help that was given (and may have been unwanted) gratefully – or even if they *are* thanked – it isn't sufficient. 'They never thank me for all I do for them' is a common complaint.

This is often a generational pattern, where the parent themself was overly responsible and the child learns to emulate this behaviour. The martyr parent is often seen as self-sacrificing, always putting the needs of others before their own. This can lead to the child feeling a sense of guilt for pursuing their own needs and desires, and they may suppress these to avoid causing any perceived inconvenience or distress to the parent.

Children of martyr parents see their parent prioritising the needs of others to their own detriment, which can lead to a skewed understanding of responsibility, where children feel compelled to take on excessive responsibilities to gain approval or avoid conflict. They often learn to anticipate the needs of others, even before they are expressed. This can lead to a pattern of over-functioning in relationships, where they take on more than their fair share of responsibilities and have difficulty asserting their own needs and desires. This pattern can continue into adulthood, setting the stage for people-pleasing and over-functioning in both personal and professional relationships.

Recognising these patterns and understanding their origins is the first step towards breaking the cycle and developing healthier relationships with responsibility and self-care. There's nothing wrong in helping others, it is both lovely to offer and receive support in this way, just as it is wonderful to receive thanks, but I guarantee that your life will get a lot better if you stop doing things with the expectation that someone will behave in the specific way that you want them to. Be honest with yourself: do you do things for the joy of helping someone or because you want the praise on the other side of it, and because it bolsters a part of your identity and how you're seen?

Pull Up

What follows is how I like to determine whether I'm being helpful and if I'm just being responsible for myself, or if I'm over-functioning and trying to do way too much for someone else (perhaps even against their wishes).

Start by picturing someone – your friend, colleague or partner – trying to climb over a garden wall, not just a piddly wall that you can step over, but one that's high enough to require effort to climb over. If I'm helping someone, I might get on my knees and hold my hands out to give them a bunk-up, just enough to get them going, and after that it's on them to get over the wall. If, on the other hand, I'm over-functioning, I'll be pushing them all the way up or on to the top of the wall trying to get them over. With the bunk-up, I'm helping them to get started. When I'm pushing, I'm putting in so much effort that I'm doing it for them and not letting them do it for themselves, which isn't helpful in the short or long term. (There are, of course, times when someone is unable to function and it's helpful and important that we step in and help.)

Over-functioning for others is an urge and, just like trying not to eat a bar of chocolate, it's very tempting to just go with the urge, especially when this is the kind of behaviour that has served you in some way in your life, or if you've been praised for it and built your identity around behaving in this way.

However, over-functioning can lead to burnout, stress and resentment. It can also hinder the growth and development of others by not allowing them the opportunity to learn and grow from their experiences. Moreover, over-functioning can lead to an imbalance in relationships, with the over-functioner often feeling unappreciated and the other party feeling overwhelmed or incompetent. Researchers have also found that over-functioning can lead to burnout in the workplace, with employees who consistently take on more tasks and responsibilities than their role requires often experiencing higher levels of job dissatisfaction and burnout.

Over-functioning in romantic relationships is common among my clients and leads to an imbalance in the relationship dynamics. It's when one partner takes on more than their fair share of responsibilities, often to the point of doing tasks that the other partner is capable of doing themselves. This can stem from a variety of factors, such as a desire to be needed, a fear of letting others down, a belief that the other partner is incapable of handling their responsibilities and what was modelled to you growing up.

My historic tendency has been to do this in romantic relationships and, while I'm glad to say that, on the whole, I have addressed this, there are times when I catch myself wanting to over-function. A few years ago, I was due to go on a nine-day work trip and my brain wanted to over-function and organise my family's time for them while I was gone. To be very clear with you, my partner does not need me to do this at all. He's perfectly capable of parenting on his own while I'm away and, in all likelihood, would much prefer me to stay out of it altogether. But my brain was telling me to organise times for our son to hang out with his friends, and that I should schedule some online food shopping deliveries, and to arrange visits to various people, and to do all these things. Thankfully, I'm skilled at noticing when I do this, so I clocked what my brain was doing and the route it was going down, and gave myself a good talking-to. I realised that I was literally heaving Paul over the wall when he hadn't even asked me to help him get over it. In his eyes there probably was no wall.

Instead, what I ended up doing was simply asking Paul, 'Is there anything we can do before I go that would help you and Nelson to have a good time together while I'm gone?' His reply was very different to what I'd come up with in my head. He responded, 'I'd love it if you and I had some time alone before you go. And it would be great if all three of us had some quality time before you leave. And I also don't think it'd be good if you're rushing to pack on the day that you leave.' Notice how he didn't need me to do any of the action items that I had come up with and how his last request was about what *I* needed to do; it had nothing to do with what *they* needed.

The flip-side of being overly responsible for others is that you're also being under-responsible for yourself. In the example above, I was focused on them, but I wasn't focused on getting my shit together before I left – I was being over-responsible for them and under-responsible for me. Thankfully, I saw what my brain was doing and I redirected it, but imagine what it would have cost me if I hadn't done that. Now apply that to a lifetime of over-functioning – no wonder so many of us are exhausted.

Allowing someone else to be responsible for themselves will require you to sit on your hands and shut your mouth, and that may feel very uncomfortable, but it's to your benefit (and probably theirs) that you stop over-functioning.

Don't Blame It On the Sunshine

A word of warning: Your brain might not like what I'm about to say, but that's okay. What I'd love you to do is notice how your brain and body respond to what I'm about to say, because that in itself is helpful. Pay attention to any defensiveness that comes up or if you find yourself arguing with me, which may happen.

Under-responsibility, or abdicating responsibility, is all about failing to fulfil a responsibility or a duty. It's about assigning responsibility to other people or to things like lack of time, the weather, your hormones or having a bad day. Now, your brain might be telling you, 'But, those things do matter,' and sometimes they really do, but let's play around with things.

Consider the scenario where you're late for a meeting at work, but instead of acknowledging that you didn't manage your time well, you blame the traffic, the alarm clock that didn't go off or, more likely, the barista who took too long with your coffee. This is a classic example of under-responsibility. You're assigning the blame to external factors instead of taking responsibility for your actions.

Or let's say you're feeling irritable and snap at a friend. Instead of apologising and acknowledging your behaviour, you blame it on your hormones or a bad day at work. While these factors can indeed influence our mood, they don't absolve us of the responsibility for how we treat others.

Now imagine that you're part of a group project at work or university and it isn't going smoothly and the deadline is looming. Instead of stepping up and contributing more, you find yourself blaming the group leader for poor organisation and delegation, your team members for their lack of effort, or even the complexity of the project itself. You might say things like, 'They should have assigned tasks more clearly,' or 'If only my team members were more competent,' or 'This project is just too complex for our timeline.' This is a classic case of under-responsibility. You're focusing on the perceived shortcomings of others or the external circumstances, rather than looking at what you could do differently.

In each of these examples, the common thread is a refusal to accept responsibility for one's actions and their consequences. Instead, the blame is shifted on to external factors or other people. While it's true that we can't control everything that happens to us, we can control how we respond, and that's where self-responsibility comes in. It's about acknowledging our role in our experiences and understanding that we have the power to influence our circumstances, rather than being passive victims of them. Here are some common ways in which we try to avoid responsibility:

Blaming others

This is a tactic where people shift the responsibility for a situation on to someone else. It's easier to point fingers at others than to accept that we may have contributed to the problem. For example, rather than admitting they didn't manage their workload effectively or communicate their needs clearly, a team member blames their missed deadline on another colleague who didn't provide information on time.

Playing the victim

In this scenario, people portray themselves as the victim, thereby absolving themselves of any responsibility for what has happened. They see themselves as having no control over the situation – like a friend who always seems to have drama in their life and blames others for their misfortunes or a colleague who constantly feels overlooked for promotions and blames their manager or colleagues for not recognising their work, instead of seeking feedback or improving their skills.

Denial

Some people simply deny their role in a situation. They refuse to acknowledge that their actions or decisions may have contributed to the problem. For example, a manager denies that their harsh communication style is causing low team morale, attributing it instead to external factors like market conditions or company policies.

Procrastination

By continually putting things off, we can avoid taking responsibility for tasks or decisions. This often leads to last-minute rushes to complete tasks, or missed deadlines and a backlog of work that impacts other team members and project timelines.

Deflection

Changing the subject or focus to avoid dealing with the issue at hand is another classic way of avoiding responsibility. When confronted about their excessive spending, someone deflects by bringing up their partner's past financial mistakes or when given feedback about their performance, an employee deflects by pointing out a mistake their supervisor made. If you're prone to falling into this trap of tit for tat, see pages 192–3.

Rationalisation

People often use rationalisation to justify their actions or decisions, even when they know they are wrong, digging themselves deeper and deeper. This is a way of avoiding responsibility by convincing themselves, and trying to persuade others, that their actions were justified. For example, a manager could justify their decision not to promote an employee by saying they're not ready, rather than admitting bias.

Passivity

Some people avoid responsibility by being overly passive and letting others make decisions for them. That way, if things go wrong, they can blame the person who made the decision instead of accepting any responsibility themselves. If they always let their partner make decisions about their shared life, from what to have for dinner to where to go on vacation, they can avoid making a wrong choice. Similarly, an employee who never voices their opinion in meetings, or takes the lead on projects, can avoid the blame if things go wrong.

The Sweet Spot of Self-responsibility

Finding the balance between over-responsibility and under-responsibility is a delicate act. It requires perspective and understanding of your role, as well as the extent of your influence in different situations. It's about acknowledging that while you have control over your actions and reactions, you cannot control everything around you. This balance is the sweet spot of self-responsibility.

When you find this sweet spot, you experience a sense of ownership over your life and experiences, even the not-so-great stuff, without blaming yourself or others, and without over-functioning for others. You're not in victim mode, making everyone else responsible for how you feel. You're not blaming others and you're not blaming yourself either. You're not people-pleasing by making yourself responsible for other people's thoughts and feelings, which are their responsibility. Instead, you're taking responsibility for everything that is yours to be responsible for.

This level of self-responsibility gives you the freedom and space to make decisions, to act and to react. It allows you to influence your future and to shape your life in the way you want it to be, and in doing so you acknowledge that you are the producer of your life circumstances, not just the product of them.

When you're self-responsible, you're able to own what's going on in your life, even the not-so-great stuff. When something undesirable happens, instead of blaming yourself or others, you approach the situation with curiosity. You ask yourself, 'How did I create this result?' This question is not about finding fault, but about understanding your role in the situation. The sweet spot of self-responsibility is not about feeling guilty or ashamed when things go wrong. It's about understanding your role, learning from your experiences, and using that knowledge to grow and evolve. It's about being proactive, self-regulating, self-reflecting and embracing your agency.

Mission Possible

Agency refers to the ability to take action or to choose what action to take. It's the sense of control you have in your life and your capacity to influence your thoughts, feelings and behaviour, which, when combined, result in you expressing your individual power. This sense of what you can do and the power to affect your future is crucial in understanding the importance of self-responsibility.

When you have little agency in your life, you believe that you don't have much control over the circumstances of your life – life happens to you and you're unable to influence it. When you exercise agency, you are essentially taking responsibility for your actions and emotional well-being. Instead of abdicating responsibility to external factors or other people, you acknowledge your power to influence your thoughts, feelings and behaviour, and therefore the outcomes in your life.

For instance, if you find yourself blaming time for not completing a task, you are abdicating responsibility to time. But it could be that you didn't plan properly, you didn't give yourself enough time or you said yes when you really meant no, leading to over-commitment. In this context, exercising agency would mean taking responsibility for your schedule and workload, and making honest decisions about what you can and cannot do.

Agency and self-responsibility go hand in hand. When you exercise agency, you are taking responsibility for your life. And the more self-responsible you are, the more resilient and courageous you will become.

Taking responsibility for your actions and outcomes is a skill that can be honed with practice. However, it's crucial to strike a balance between being responsible and over-responsible. When something undesirable happens, instead of blaming yourself or others, approach the situation with curiosity. Ask yourself, 'How did I contribute to this result?' This question isn't about self-blame, but about understanding your role in the situation. People who perceive themselves as having personal control over their environment are more likely to take responsibility for their actions. This sense of control, or perceived control, is a crucial factor in taking responsibility without becoming over-responsible.

However, it's equally important to ask the same question when something desirable happens and to understand how you contributed to a positive outcome. This understanding allows you to replicate positive results in the future. Attributing positive outcomes solely to external factors, like having a good day or being in the right mood, can prevent you from recognising your role in creating these outcomes. Those who attribute their successes to their own efforts and abilities, rather than external factors, are more likely to take responsibility for their actions.

Taking responsibility is a skill and if you practise this you will get more and more positive results in your life, I promise. But it's not just about creating the life you want or achieving your goals. This is about improving the process to get there, too, because when you're being self-responsible, you're not living in the extremes of being overly responsible or abdicating responsibility. You're living in the middle and it will feel powerful and solid. It doesn't mean everything will be rosy all the time – that's not the point and it's not achievable – but you won't be blaming yourself, blaming others or blaming life.

You also won't be overly concerned with things that have nothing to do with you and are not your responsibility. I want you to imagine for a moment how much energy and mental space this will save you. How much more sleep you'll get. How it will free you up to problem-solve from your highest ability, because you're rooted in being responsible. How it will influence your relationships and your work life. I am telling you – self-responsibility is where it's at.

EPILOGUE: THE JOURNEY HOME

Coming home isn't always about a physical location. True homecoming is an inner journey into yourself. Throughout this book, we've navigated complex terrains, from the nuances of the nervous system to all the thoughts your brain comes up with, but the culmination of this journey is in arriving in that intimate space within yourself where you truly accept and embrace yourself.

Feeling at home in your body and mind isn't a concept – it's a profound sense of grounding. It's the feeling you get when you shut the door, take a deep breath and realise you're in a place of safety, understanding and acceptance. Only in this case, that door isn't to a house or a room, it's who you are, and it's in this place that you meet your most powerful self. A settled strength emanates from this place and it's the power of knowing who you are, accepting every facet of yourself with compassion, and realising that every experience, emotion and thought has its rightful place.

As you move forward, remember that this place is always accessible to you. When the world feels chaotic or when doubt creeps in, come home to yourself. Remind yourself of your journey, your discoveries and the home you've built within. This is where you'll find your true power – power that's rooted in self-awareness, acceptance and love.

ACKNOWLEDGEMENTS

To my coach and dear friend Robin Langford, who told me that I would write this book long before I was willing to consider that I would, and who helped me in innumerable ways throughout the process. I am so thankful for all your insights, wisdom, coaching and friendship.

Thanks to Bev Aron, who casually mentioned that I could write this book far quicker than I was expecting and with greater ease. The possibility that you offered me planted a seed and set the tone for how I would approach writing this time around. Thank you to Stacey Boehman, for asking me the one question that made me realise I didn't want to write the book that I originally set out to write. That moment of coaching resulted in me taking a year off from anything to do with books and it was that space that led to this book coming out of me.

Thank you to my agent Julia Silk, for championing me and my ideas so fervently, for all the nudges to reply to the emails that I forget about and get buried in my inbox, and for suggesting that this was the book for me to write.

Thank you to Charlotte Croft at Green Tree, for understanding that I needed time away from writing books and for jumping on board with my plan for this one. We've birthed three books together now, and I'm endlessly grateful for your keen editing skills, staunch belief in me and for our relationship. Thank you to Sarah Skipper, for your helpful questions and skilful editing, and to Sarah Head, Lizzy Ewer and Katherine Macpherson for your individual contributions and collective support that I am eternally grateful for.

A huge thank you to my team: Bek, Robyn, Casey and Amy. There is no way I could simultaneously run my business and write a book without your help. Who you all are and how you work is what's enabled me to switch off and write, and I am so grateful to have such incredible women working with me and helping my clients.

Where would I be without my amazing coach mates? Mars Lord, Vikki Louise, Becca Pike, Maggie Reyes, Victoria Albina, Erica Reitman and Leona Baker. The conversations we have always light me up and regardless of how little I see of you (some of you I've known for years and am still to meet in person) I feel surrounded and held by your love. Thank you to Fabeku for the sessions we had together while I was going through a significant identity shift – what was uncovered during those sessions continues to breathe and evolve.

And then there's the Margate lot: Harriet and Meghan, Natalie, Naomi, Natalie and Alex, Emma and Ian, Scott and Helina. Thank you to the whole crew at Forts Margate. The majority of this book was written at table 3 and occasionally at table 7. You not only kept me going with delicious filter coffee, toasties and French toast, but with your friendly faces, great chat and contributions when I wanted an opinion on something. And thank you to Julia, Casey and the team at Nelson Park Riding Centre – learning to horse ride with you has changed my life in so many ways, including time every week when I couldn't think about the book, because all my attention was on staying on your horses!

To my mum and dad for giving birth to not one but two absolute legends. I'm so glad that I got you both as parents and that I had the good fortune to end up with Sam as a brother. Mum, you're not here to read this, but it's important to me to acknowledge your presence within the chapters – you did a great job of raising me, thank you. Dad, thank you for always acknowledging my efforts, strengths and successes, and for celebrating with me. I know now how many people don't receive that from either parent, let alone both.

Thank you to Sam and Sandra. Sam, you are my brother, friend and now colleague too. To my son, Nelson, thank you for (mostly) not disturbing me when I was working on a chapter and not watching TV and playing football with you (and thank you for all the snuggles you did disturb me with). Thank you to Paul, for being such a willing partner in this escapade and all the others, for ensuring that I could work throughout weekends when I was in the flow and for teaching me how to approach life differently. Thank you for being my safe place.

REFERENCES

Chapter 1: Staying alive

'there is a mounting body of evidence that shows that stress *does* have negative consequences for our health and well-being': Yaribeygi, H., Panahi, Y., Sahraei, H., Johnston, T. P. and Sahebkar, A. The impact of stress on body function: A review. EXCLI J. 2017 Jul 21;16:1057-1072. doi: 10.17179/excli2017-480. PMID: 28900385; PMCID: PMC5579396.

'(there's also evidence that says it really depends on how you frame the stress)': Keller, A., Litzelman, K., Wisk, L. E., Maddox, T., Cheng, E. R., Creswell, P. D., and Witt, W. P., Does the perception that stress affects health matter? The association with health and mortality. *Health Psychol.* 2012 Sep;31(5):677-84. doi: 10.1037/a0026743. Epub 2011 Dec 26. PMID: 22201278; PMCID: PMC3374921.; McGonigal, K. (2015). *The upside of stress: why stress is good for you, and how to get good at it.* Avery.

'it is now generally accepted that the amygdala plays a significant role in creating emotional responses': Janak, P. H. and Tye, K. M., From circuits to behaviour in the amygdala. *Nature.* 2015 Jan 15;517(7534):284-92. doi: 10.1038/nature14188. PMID: 25592533; PMCID: PMC4565157.

'In 2017, a Swedish study found that 69.8 per cent of women who had experienced sexual assault reported experiencing tonic immobility.': Möller A, Söndergaard HP, Helström L. Tonic immobility during sexual assault - a common reaction predicting post-traumatic stress disorder and severe depression. Acta Obstet Gynecol Scand. 2017 Aug;96(8):932-938. doi: 10.1111/aogs.13174. Epub 2017 Jun 22. PMID: 28589545.

'Polyvagal theory', 'In his proposed theory, Porges states that the SES emerged as the brain and cranial nerves developed': Porges SW. The polyvagal perspective. *Biol Psychol.* 2007 Feb;74(2):116-43. doi: 10.1016/j.biopsycho.2006.06.009. Epub 2006 Oct 16. PMID: 17049418; PMCID: PMC1868418.

'Stress can impact the structure and functioning of these neural loops and pathways.': McEwen, B. S., Nasca, G. and Gray, J.D., Stress Effects on Neuronal Structure: Hippocampus, Amygdala, and Prefrontal Cortex. *Neuropsychopharmacology.* 2016 Jan;41(1):3-23. doi: 10.1038/npp.2015.171. Epub 2015 Jun 16. PMID: 26076834; PMCID: PMC4677120.

References

'Studies have revealed that chronic stress can lead to increased amygdala activity': Shin, L. M. and Liberzon, I., The neurocircuitry of fear, stress, and anxiety disorders. *Neuropsychopharmacology.* 2010 Jan;35(1):169-91. doi: 10.1038/npp.2009.83. PMID: 19625997; PMCID: PMC3055419.
'Chronic stress has been found to impair the prefrontal cortex's ability to regulate emotional responses effectively': Arnsten, A. F. Stress signalling pathways that impair prefrontal cortex structure and function. *Nat Rev Neurosci.* 2009 Jun;10(6):410-22. doi: 10.1038/nrn2648. PMID: 19455173; PMCID: PMC2907136.
'researchers have found evidence of neural plasticity': Khalsa, D. S. Stress, Meditation, and Alzheimer's Disease Prevention: Where The Evidence Stands. *J Alzheimers Dis.* 2015;48(1):1-12. doi: 10.3233/JAD-142766. PMID: 26445019; PMCID: PMC4923750.
'Studies have highlighted the positive impact of physical exercise': Mandolesi, L., Polverino, A., Montuori, S., Foti, F., Ferraioli, G., Sorrentino, P., and Sorrentino, G., Effects of Physical Exercise on Cognitive Functioning and Wellbeing: Biological and Psychological Benefits. *Front Psychol.* 2018 Apr 27;9:509. doi: 10.3389/fpsyg.2018.00509. PMID: 29755380; PMCID: PMC5934999.
'Research conducted by Dr Rachel Yehuda and her colleagues examined the descendants of Holocaust survivors and found alterations in stress hormone regulation and increased prevalence of stress-related disorders': Yehuda, R. and Lehrner, A. Intergenerational transmission of trauma effects: putative role of epigenetic mechanisms. *World Psychiatry.* 2018 Oct;17(3):243-257. doi: 10.1002/wps.20568. PMID: 30192087; PMCID: PMC6127768.

Chapter 2: Procrastination

'Researchers Dianne Tice and Ellen Bratslavsky encapsulated this phenomenon in the phrase "giving in to feel good"': Tice, D. M. and Bratslavsky, E. (2000). Giving in to Feel Good: The Place of Emotion Regulation in the Context of General Self-Control. Psychological Inquiry, 11(3), 149–159. Available from http://www.jstor.org/stable/1449793.
'affecting up to 30 per cent of the population, with a higher prevalence among women': Frost, R. O., Marten, P., Lahart, C. and Rosenblate, R. (1990). The dimensions of perfectionism. *Cognitive Therapy and Research*, 14(5), 449–468. 10.1007/BF01172967.
'poor executive functioning skills, which is linked with autism and ADHD.': Otterman, D. L., Koopman-Verhoeff, M.E., White, T. J., Tiemeier, H., Bolhuis, K. and Jansen, P.W., Executive functioning and neurodevelopmental

disorders in early childhood: a prospective population-based study. *Child Adolesc Psychiatry Ment Health*. 2019 Oct 22;13:38. doi: 10.1186/s13034-019-0299-7. PMID: 31649749; PMCID: PMC6805591.

'Stress impairs executive function': Zareyan, S., Zhang, H., Wang, J., Song, W., Hampson, E., Abbott, D. and Diamond, A., First Demonstration of Double Dissociation between COMT-Met158 and COMT-Val158 Cognitive Performance When Stressed and When Calmer. Cereb Cortex. 2021 Feb 5;31(3):1411-1426. doi: 10.1093/cercor/bhaa276. PMID: 33124661; PMCID: PMC8599760.

'mindful movement activities such as traditional martial arts, qi gong, tai qi and yoga have been shown to enhance executive functioning': Lakes, K. D. and Hoyt, W. T. (2004). Promoting self-regulation through school-based martial arts training. *J. Appl. Dev. Psychol*. 25 283–302.

Ren, F. F., Chen, F. T., Zhou, W. S., Cho, Y. M., Ho, T. J., Hung, T. M. and Chang, Y. K., Effects of Chinese Mind-Body Exercises on Executive Function in Middle-Aged and Older Adults: A Systematic Review and Meta-Analysis. *Front Psychol*. 2021 May 21; 12:656141. doi: 10.3389/fpsyg.2021.656141. PMID: 34093345; PMCID: PMC8175659, and Gothe, N. P., Keswani, R. K. and McAuley, E., Yoga practice improves executive function by attenuating stress levels. *Biol Psychol*. 2016 Dec;121(Pt A):109-116. doi: 10.1016/j.biopsycho.2016.10.010. Epub 2016 Oct 26. PMID: 27794449.

'the idea behind temptation bundling': Milkman, K. L., Minson, J. A. and Volpp, K. G., Holding the Hunger Games Hostage at the Gym: An Evaluation of Temptation Bundling. *Manage Sci*. 2014 Feb;60(2):283-299. doi: 10.1287/mnsc.2013.1784. PMID: 25843979; PMCID: PMC4381662.

'In a research study conducted by Milkman': Milkman, K.L., Minson, J.A., Volpp, K.G., Holding the Hunger Games Hostage at the Gym: An Evaluation of Temptation Bundling. *Manage Sci*. 2014 Feb;60(2):283-299. doi: 10.1287/mnsc.2013.1784. PMID: 25843979; PMCID: PMC4381662, https://www.ncbi.nlm.nih.gov/pmc/articles/PMC4381662.

Chapter 3: Defensiveness

'This term, coined by professor of psychiatry, Dr Dan Siegel, refers to the zone of arousal in which a person can function most effectively.': Siegel, Daniel J., 1957-. (1999). The developing mind: toward a neurobiology of interpersonal experience. New York: Guilford Press.

'Centers for Disease Control (CDC) and Kaiser Permanente healthcare organisation in California.': Felitti, V. J., Anda, R. F., Nordenberg, D., Williamson, D. F., Spitz, A. M., Edwards, V., Koss, M. P. and Marks, J. S.,

Relationship of childhood abuse and household dysfunction to many of the leading causes of death in adults. The Adverse Childhood Experiences (ACE) Study. Am J Prev Med. 1998 May;14(4):245-58. doi: 10.1016/s0749-3797(98)00017-8. PMID: 9635069.

'In a 2014 UK study on ACEs, 47 per cent of people had experienced at least one ACE': Bellis, M. A., Hughes, K., Leckenby, N., Perkins, C. and Lowey, H., National household survey of adverse childhood experiences and their relationship with resilience to health-harming behaviors in England. BMC Med. 2014 May 2;12:72. doi: 10.1186/1741-7015-12-72. PMID: 24886026; PMCID: PMC4234527.

Chapter 5: People-pleasing

'Fawning (also known as please-and-appease), was coined by psychotherapist Pete Walker,': Walker, P. (2013). *Complex PTSD: from surviving to thriving: a guide and map for recovering from childhood trauma.* First Edition. Lafayette, CA, Azure Coyote.

'Ask for Angela': https://www.met.police.uk/police-forces/metropolitan-police/areas/about-us/about-the-met/campaigns/ask-for-angela.

Chapter 6: Emotions

'Toxic positivity refers to the overzealous application of happiness and optimism': https://www.psychologytoday.com/gb/Basics/toxic-positivity.

'There is a principle known as Hebb's rule, which states that when neurons fire at the same time, the connections between them strengthen': Hebb, D. O. (1949). *The Organisation of Behaviour.* New York, NY: John Wiley & Sons.

'This is a basic form of associative learning and it's the foundation of classical conditioning, a concept introduced by Russian physiologist Ivan Pavlov.': Pavlov, I. P. (1927) *Conditioned Reflexes: An Investigation of the Physiological Activity of the Cerebral Cortex.* Translated and Edited by G. V. Anrep. Oxford University Press, London, 142.

'The theory of emotion, proposed in 1884 by psychologists William James and Carl Lange, suggests that our emotional experiences are reactions to physiological changes in our bodies.': James, W. (1884). What is an emotion? *Mind, 9,* 188–205.

'The two-factor theory, also known as the Schachter-Singer theory, suggests that our emotions come from both our body's physiological reaction and how our mind interprets those reactions.': Schachter, S. and Singer, J.E.,

Cognitive, social, and physiological determinants of emotional state. *Psychol Rev.* 1962 Sep; 69:379-99. doi: 10.1037/h0046234. PMID: 14497895. 'Research has also shown that improving interoceptive awareness can enhance the intensity of emotional experiences and improve emotional regulation.': Tan, Y., Wang, X., Blain, S. D., Jia, L. and Qui, J., Interoceptive attention facilitates emotion regulation strategy use. *Int J Clin Health Psychol.* 2023 Jan-Apr;23(1):100336. doi: 10.1016/j.ijchp.2022.100336. Epub 2022 Sep 22. PMID: 36199366; PMCID: PMC9512845.

'Alexithymia, a term coined by Dr Peter Sifneos in 1972, describes a unique emotional experience where an individual struggles to identify and articulate their emotions.': Sifneos, P. E., Alexithymia, clinical issues, politics and crime. *Psychother Psychosom.* 2000 May–Jun;69(3):113-6. doi: 10.1159/000012377. PMID: 10877675.

'About 10 per cent of the population experience alexithymia to a high degree.': Franz, M., Popp, K., Schaefer, R., Sitte, W., Schneider, C., Hardt, J., Decker, O. and Braehler, E. Alexithymia in the German general population. *Soc Psychiatry Psychiatr Epidemiol.* 2008 Jan;43(1):54-62. doi: 10.1007/s00127-007-0265-1. Epub 2007 Oct 12. PMID: 17934682.

'researchers have identified two aspects of alexithymia': Vorst, H. C. M. and Bermond, B. (2001): Validity and reliability of the Bermond-Vorst Alexithymia Questionnaire. *Pers Individ Dif* 30:413–434.

'Research suggests that synaesthesia might be due to increased connectivity or communication between different areas of the brain': Brang, D. and Ramachandran, V. S., Survival of the synesthesia gene: why do people hear colors and taste words? PLoS Biol. 2011 Nov;9(11):e1001205. doi: 10.1371/journal.pbio.1001205. Epub 2011 Nov 22. PMID: 22131906; PMCID: PMC3222625.

'But research has shown that social support and co-regulation can have a significant impact on mental health': Harandi, T. F., Taghinasab, M. M. and Nayeri, T. D., The correlation of social support with mental health: A meta-analysis. *Electron Physician.* 2017 Sep 25;9(9):5212-5222. doi: 10.19082/5212. PMID: 29038699; PMCID: PMC5633215.

Chapter 7: Decisions

'Welcome to the paradox of choice': Schwartz, Barry, 1946-. The Paradox of Choice: Why More Is Less. New York :Ecco, 2004.

'Cognitive dissonance is a theory that was proposed by Leon Festinger in 1957': Festinger, L. (1957). An Introduction to the Theory of Dissonance. In L. Festinger (ed.), A Theory of Cognitive Dissonance (pp. 1–30). Stanford, CA: Stanford University Press.

'This aligns with the concept of "affective forecasting" proposed by psychologists Timothy Wilson and Daniel Gilbert, which suggests that we're often inaccurate in predicting our future emotional state': Wilson, T. D. and Gilbert, D. T. (2003). Affective forecasting. *Advances in Experimental Social Psychology*, 35, 345–411.

'The concept was popularised by social psychologist Roy F. Baumeister and is based on the Freudian hypothesis of ego depletion': Baumeister, Roy F. (2003), 'The Psychology of Irrationality', in Brocas, Isabelle; Carrillo, Juan D. (eds.), *The Psychology of Economic Decisions: Rationality and Well-being*, pp. 1–15, ISBN 978-0-19-925108-7.

'This reframing technique is backed by research in cognitive psychology, which shows that how we frame or interpret situations can significantly impact our emotional and behavioural responses': Kross, E. and Ayduk, O. (2017). Self-Distancing: Theory, Research, and Current Directions. *Advances in Experimental Social Psychology*, 55, 81–136.

'Research has shown that our brains are wired to seek certainty and avoid uncertainty. A study by University College London.': de Berker, A. O., Rutledge, R. B., Mathys, C., Marshall, L., Cross, G. F., Dolan, R. J. and Bestmann, S., Computations of uncertainty mediate acute stress responses in humans. Nat Commun. 2016 Mar 29;7:10996. doi: 10.1038/ncomms10996. PMID: 27020312; PMCID: PMC4820542.

'Research has shown that people who are comfortable with uncertainty are less likely to fall into cognitive biases, such as overconfidence or confirmation bias, and are more likely to be creative and innovative': Sorrentino, R. M., Roney, C. J., Hanna, S. E. and Nezlek, J. B. (2017). Uncertainty orientation and affective experiences: Individual differences in reactions to situations of high and low uncertainty. *Journal of Personality and Social Psychology*, 113(4), 513–524.

'Research has shown that self-trust is associated with a range of positive outcomes': Rotter, J. B. (1967). A new scale for the measurement of interpersonal trust. *Journal of Personality*, 35(4), 651–665, and Mischel, W. (1977). The interaction of person and situation. In D. Magnusson & N. S. Endler (eds.), Personality at the crossroads: Current issues in interactional psychology (pp. 333–352). Lawrence Erlbaum.

Chapter 9: Hard conversations

'Researchers simulated the experience of rejection by asking people who had recently experienced an unwanted breakup to look at a photograph of their ex-partner': Kross, E., Berman, M. G., Mischel, W., Smith, E. E. and Wager, T. D., Social rejection shares somatosensory representations with physical pain. Proc Natl Acad Sci U S A. 2011 Apr 12;108(15):6270-5. doi: 10.1073/pnas.1102693108. Epub 2011 Mar 28. PMID: 21444827; PMCID: PMC3076808.

'We've established that rejection doesn't feel good, but some experts suspect that it is an even more intense experience for some individuals': Dodson, W. W. How ADHD Ignites Rejection Sensitive Dysphoria (https://www .additudemag .com /rejection -sensitive -dysphoria -and -adhd/). *ADDitude*. 2017, 7 Feb.

'*Psychology Today* highlights that because it doesn't "officially" exist as a condition, there is no quantifiable criteria that can be used to establish if an individual has RSD or not': https://www .psychologytoday .com /gb /basics / rejection-sensitivity.

Chapter 10: Self-responsibility

'Researchers have also found that over-functioning can lead to burnout in the workplace': Bakker, A. B., Demerouti, E. and Sanz-Vergel, A. I. (2014). Burnout and work engagement: The JD–R approach. *Annual Review of Organizational Psychology and Organizational Behavior*, 1, 389–411.

'However, over-functioning can lead to burnout, stress and resentment': Skowron, E. A. and Friedlander, M. L. (1998). The Differentiation of Self Inventory: Development and initial validation. *Journal of Counseling Psychology*, 45(3), 235–246.

'Researchers have also found that over-functioning can lead to burnout in the workplace': Bakker, A. B., Demerouti, E. and Sanz-Vergel, A. I. (2014). Burnout and work engagement: The JD–R approach. *Annual Review of Organizational Psychology and Organizational Behavior*, 1, 389–411.

INDEX

Index

Index